# TAKE CONTROL OF YOUR HEART DISEASE RISK

JOHN WHYTE, MD, MPH

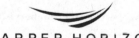

HARPER HORIZON

## TO EMILIO

Thank you for giving us tools to find our purpose.

An ounce of PREVENTION

is worth a pound of CURE.

—BENJAMIN FRANKLIN

# CONTENTS

# FOREWORD

DR. PHIL MCGRAW

ONE PERSON DIES FROM HEART DISEASE every minute in America. It is the leading cause of death, with 650,000 people lost in 2020.

Heart disease is caused by many factors, including family history, poor diet, and lack of physical activity. But there is more—even ancient literature acknowledged the role of emotions. The Greek poet Homer wrote of a character in *The Odyssey* who spoke of dying of a broken heart. Yet centuries later many people don't seem to focus on the fact that our emotions really do and always have played a key role in many aspects of heart disease.

This lack of awareness is despite the wealth of data in recent years that shows the relationship between our emotional health and our heart health is so much more than a poetic metaphor. Study after study demonstrates that anger, stress, depression, and even loneliness and anxiety cause biochemical changes that translate to physiologic alterations in our hearts. We know that chronic stress influences how well our blood vessels clot, and overwhelming depression can literally alter the shape of our hearts. Yet many people still possess a mindset that emotions don't play a role in our overall health. As a result, we tend to dismiss them when thinking about our health. We think that things will just get better, particularly if we ignore them. What's striking is that we often recognize the impact mental health has on others but often ignore it in ourselves. Too often doctors will similarly ignore the mental and emotional adjustment of a patient in making diagnoses and formulating treatment plans.

We need a new mindset that acknowledges that physical health and mental health are inextricably linked. Most doctors are certainly aware of the powerful mind-body connection, but dealing with it can be time consuming, awkward, and outside of their comfort zone. Even broaching the subject with patients who are seeking treatment for what they conceptualize as a one-dimensional "physical" ailment can often result in their being defensive or resistant to such dialogue. As a result, health-care professionals often don't talk enough about this in a meaningful way and often aren't skilled at explaining *why* it's important. Many patients leave the office confused, wondering why they're being counseled about their mood when they came to talk about their blood pressure and cholesterol level.

That's why I am so pleased that Dr. John Whyte is not a physician who merely treats a disease, a disorder, or an organ—Dr. Whyte treats the *entire integrated patient.*

Quite naturally he addresses both physical and mental components of heart disease in his book *Take Control of Your Heart Disease Risk.* The good doctor *always* writes about things that matter to people who care. That is why Robin and I have read everything he has written.

There are many books that offer accurate advice on what to eat and how to exercise. But that information, however accurate, is like giving the reader half of a treasure map! Dr. Whyte goes several steps further, detailing the scientific relationship between how we feel and how our hearts functions. He explains *how to recognize* anxiety and depression as well as chronic stress—and, more importantly, *what to do about it*. We desperately need to be having these discussions around the mind-body connection in a way that empowers people to take charge of their lives. Dr. Whyte is a pioneer in leading the charge, and his book can set in motion a zeitgeist for refreshing our thinking and taking an evidence-based approach to heart disease.

Maximizing your mental and emotional health must be a part of your personal risk reduction strategy. As someone who has been on the television in many of your homes for more than two decades, I know well the impact mental health exacts on individuals as well as their families. I also know the role it plays when it comes to heart disease, and so does my dear friend and colleague Dr. Whyte. That is why I asked for the privilege of writing the foreword to this important and life-saving book. Dr. Whyte is giving us the rest of the map, and I believe the wisdom in these pages will have a profound impact in the fight against heart disease. You are the most important member of *your* treatment team, and you are about to be empowered by Dr. John Whyte to take control of your heart disease risk.

"Dr. Phil" McGraw
September 2022

# INTRODUCTION

## HOW'S MY HEART?

It's a question patients often ask me. Sometimes they phrase it in a more fun way: "How's my ticker, Doc?"

I know what they mean. They want to know if they are going to die from heart disease. Of course, I can't predict the future, but thanks to new tools, I can help them estimate their risk of a heart attack in the next five to ten years.

Heart disease remains a leading cause of death. Even though we have made tremendous advances in the diagnosis and treatment of a heart attack, someone dies every minute.

What I find particularly concerning is that silent heart attacks make up more than 40 percent of all heart attacks. That means you have no symptoms. Even worse, it triples your chance of dying. Simply put—the first symptom can be fatal.

But I do have some good news. Heart disease doesn't happen overnight. It takes years to develop, and that gives you time to get it diagnosed, treated, reversed, or, better yet, prevented! That's also because most heart problems are not caused by genetics. Nearly 80 percent of heart disease is caused by lifestyle—e.g., what we eat, how active we are, the amount of stress in our lives. People are always surprised by that number. "Really, Dr. Whyte? That much. Are you sure?" is the typical response. Yes, I'm sure about the role of lifestyle, and you will be too after reading this book.

What I've also learned over twenty-five years of practice is that many people think they aren't at risk for heart disease—and therefore don't make any lifestyle changes. "Everything seems fine. I don't have any pain." They mistakenly believe that it's mostly family history, or they're too young or too busy to worry about it now. Or for some reason, they don't believe they will be affected despite recent trends. I want to change this belief, because even though the heart is powerful, we need to take care of it. Right now, most of us aren't doing as good a job as we should.

Since 2010, the American Heart Association has looked at several components to address heart health. These include diet, physical activities, nicotine exposure, blood pressure, blood sugar, cholesterol levels, and weight. In its last report published in 2022, only 7 percent of Americans met criteria for good heart health! And the trend has been getting worse for the last five years. Blood pressure control has declined, while cholesterol levels have increased. Most of us are gaining weight, with a dramatic increase in diabetes. And it's affecting younger people more often.

It doesn't have to be this way. You have the power to take control of your risk. Over the next few chapters, I will tell you what to eat, how much exercise you need to do, and how to reduce stress and improve mood, as well as what supplements or medications you need to be on or possibly stop taking. This advice can reduce risk up to 80 percent for many people.

For those of you who are at low risk today, that is great. But remember, risk changes over time, especially as we age, so adopting and maintaining healthy habits is important at any age or current risk level.

Let's go from "I hope I don't have a heart attack"—and let's be honest, we all hope that—to "How can I prevent a heart attack?" You need the tools and the strategies to help you do that. The following chapters provide what you require.

Let's get started.

## CHAPTER ONE

# What Exactly Is Heart Disease?

---

**TRUE OR FALSE?**

1. Heart disease kills more Americans every year than cancer and diabetes combined.
2. Someone dies of a heart attack every minute.
3. Sixty percent of Americans have heart disease.
4. Plaque in blood vessels can cause blockage in heart vessels.
5. Arteries carry oxygen to the heart.

*(Answers at end of chapter)*

---

HEART ATTACKS REMAIN THE NUMBER one killer in the US. One American dies every minute from heart disease. You read that correctly. Over 650,000 people die each year of a heart attack. That's one out of every four deaths. It's also the leading cause of death globally. Nearly twenty million deaths around the world are attributed to heart disease yearly. Many other people get newly diagnosed with heart disease, and the impact on their quality of life is significant.

You may be thinking, *But don't we have better treatments nowadays?* Yes, that's true. Mortality from heart disease is decreasing—certainly from a first heart attack. However, the number of people experiencing heart disease is increasing. Currently, about 30 percent of Americans have heart disease, and things aren't getting better. The American Heart Association estimates that by 2030, more than 40 percent of Americans will have some form of heart disease. That is a staggering statistic!

Let me put it in perspective this way: If recent trends continue, it's estimated that two out of three men and one out of two women will develop heart disease in their lifetimes. What's even more troubling is that when women have a heart attack, they often aren't treated as aggressively. The same is true for Blacks and Hispanics, irrespective of gender.

It may seem like heart attacks occur randomly or out of nowhere. We all have heard of someone seemingly in perfect health who died from a heart attack. For most people, though, a heart attack is not random. Heart damage typically occurs over many years, a result of a combination of genetics and lifestyle. As I mentioned earlier, recent research suggests that for most people, genetic factors make up less than 20 percent of the risk of heart disease. The rest, around 80 percent, is caused by lifestyle—primarily the quality and quantity of our food, the amount of daily physical activity we engage in, the quality of our nightly sleep, and how much chronic stress we experience. That can be scary, but, in a way, it's actually good news—because you can control much of your heart disease risk. Even though genetic factors do play a role in heart disease, recent research suggests that lifestyle often trumps genetics or at least lessens its impact. Lifestyle plays a much bigger role, so changes you make to the way you live can significantly impact whether and when you get heart disease.

## How Does the Heart Function?

The heart has so much significance to us. It represents love and life. We talk about kind people who have "big hearts" or "hearts of gold" and about mean people who are "heartless." Some people might say the brain is the most important organ, but I think it's the heart. Show a video of a beating heart and we are all in awe!

I don't want to give you an anatomy lesson in this book, but as we talk about ways to reduce your personal risk of heart disease, it's a good idea to learn what the heart looks like and what it does.

The heart has four chambers. Think of them as rooms (from the French word for chamber, meaning room). They're similar on the left and the right. The two on the top are the atria, and the two on the bottom are ventricles. One of the reasons the heart is so important for life is the role it plays in delivering oxygen. Oxygen-rich blood from your lungs flows to the left atrium, then to the left ventricle, which pumps it out to your body. Blood returns to the right atrium, then the right ventricle, which sends it back to your lungs for more oxygen. It's an intricate, fine-tuned circuit that doesn't like disruptions.

The heart isn't as big as people may think. It's the size of your fist and weighs about ten to twelve ounces. Despite its size, the heart is a powerhouse. It beats (expands and contracts) approximately one hundred thousand times per day, pumping over two thousand gallons per day, five to six quarts per minute. (The average heart rate for most adults is around seventy-five beats per minute.) Imagine doing that for your car at the gas station! It's a lot of work.

Your heart is a key part of your cardiovascular system. You'll hear that word a lot—*cardio* (heart) *vascular* (blood supply). When it comes to our blood supply, there are two main blood vessels that are part of the circuit I mentioned.

**Arteries.** These begin with the aorta, the largest artery leaving the heart. Arteries carry blood full of oxygen away from the heart to all of the cells throughout your body. They branch several times, becoming smaller and smaller as they carry blood farther from the heart and into organs. When you feel your pulse at your wrist, that's your radial artery; and when you feel it in your neck, it's your carotid artery. If you push hard in your groin area, you can feel your femoral artery.

**Veins.** These are blood vessels that take blood back to the heart. This blood has lower oxygen content and is rich in waste products that are being removed, from the body. Veins become larger and larger as they get closer to the heart. As we get older, we sometimes see these blue lines near our skin—those are our veins. And when you get blood drawn, they are using your veins.

A little fun fact: This vast system of blood vessels is over sixty thousand miles long. That's long enough to go around the world more than twice!

The term *heart disease* comprises a variety of conditions. In this book, it primarily refers to heart attacks. But there are many diseases of the heart.

Some of the most common are as follows:

**Arrhythmia.** You may have had the feeling where your heart flutters or skips a beat. That's caused by a change in your heart's rhythm—called arrhythmia. Your heartbeat is controlled by short bursts of electricity, and a minor change in those bursts typically isn't a problem. But more serious arrhythmia can keep your heart from performing its job the way it needs to, and that can cause serious problems.

If those electrical bursts really get knocked off course, you feel it—your heart may start to race or beat slower than normal. Some people might feel as if their heart vibrates. When this abnormal heart rhythm occurs, your organs and muscles may not get enough oxygen. You could have chest pain and feel lightheaded, and you might even faint. If the rhythm gets totally out of whack, your heart gets like gelatin; it quivers and can't pump at all. This is called fibrillation, and it can be life-threatening, since it can make clots go to blood vessels in your brain and heart. Atrial fibrillation (afib) is more well known nowadays, since many smartwatches can measure your heart rhythm and check for afib.

**Cardiomyopathy.** This is a group of diseases that make your heart muscle thick, stiff, or larger than usual. Getting bigger in this situation is not better. Over time, your heart gets weaker, and it's harder for it to pump blood and keep its regular rhythm. There are three main types: dilated, ischemic, and restrictive, with dilated the most common. It typically occurs in the bigger chambers of the heart, such as the left ventricle. As it gets worse, the ventricle can't pump very well, and blood starts to collect or pool in your heart.

**Heart infections.** Just as you can get infections in your lungs or your urinary tract, as two examples, you also can get an infection in your heart. As in other parts of your body, germs like bacteria or viruses and even fungi can cause an infection in different parts of your heart. Infections can be very serious and often require medications or even surgery.

**Heart valve disease.** The heart valves that guide your blood through your heart are essentially flaps that open and close with each heartbeat. This is what makes the *lub-DUB* sound of your heart. Any damage to the shape or function of a valve could make it hard to open and close the right way. When that happens, often your doctor will hear a murmur, which is a whooshing or swishing sound between heartbeats. Valve problems can make your heart work harder and cause blood flow problems: your blood flow could be blocked or narrowed (called stenosis) or blood can leak and flow backward (called regurgitation).

## ANATOMY OF THE HEART

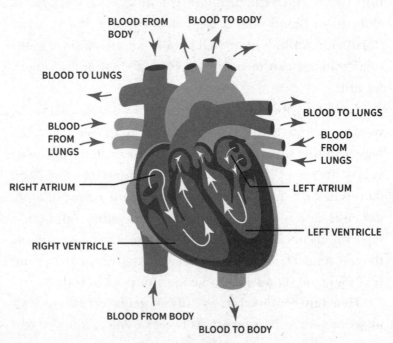

**Heart failure.** This term can be scary. It doesn't mean your heart has "failed," or stopped working. It means your heart doesn't pump as strongly as it should and therefore doesn't meet your body's needs. Typically, this causes your body to hold in salt and water, which will give you swelling and shortness of breath. Heart failure is one of the most common reasons people are admitted to the hospital—and readmitted—as they get older.

**Coronary heart disease/heart attacks.** Also called coronary artery disease, coronary heart disease is the most common type of heart disease in the US. (It's almost redundant calling it coronary, which means "heart," and then saying *heart*!) When you have it, a waxy substance called plaque builds up in your heart's arteries. You won't know it's there at first, but over time, it narrows your arteries, like a clog in a pipe. That narrowing limits the amount of blood flowing to your heart. Heart attacks occur when a break or rupture develops in a plaque. A blood clot forms at the site of the rupture and completely blocks the blood supply to a segment of the heart. If the blockage persists for more than twenty minutes, that portion of the heart muscle usually suffers irreversible damage.

In this book, I am primarily discussing your risk for heart attacks. The advice may help with some other heart conditions, partly because the strategies used to prevent heart attacks can also help reduce risk of other heart problems.

## Summary

You are more likely to die from heart disease than any other condition. Nearly a third of Americans have heart disease, and that percentage is increasing, with more young people also developing it. Learning a bit about how the heart works helps you understand what you can do—what you need to do—to develop your personal heart disease prevention program.

## ANSWERS

1. **True**. Heart disease remains the number one killer of Americans. You are more likely to die from heart disease than any other health condition.

2. **True**. A heart attack kills someone every minute.

3. **False**. Currently 40 percent of Americans have heart disease, but that number is increasing.

4. **True**. Plaque in our blood vessels can cause a blockage— just like in a pipe—preventing blood flow and oxygen to the body.

5. **False**. Arteries carry oxygen-rich blood away from the heart.

## CHAPTER TWO

# Knowing the Risks

SALLY IS FIFTY-FIVE YEARS OLD and loves baking. She's quite good at it, creating delicious treats over the years. All that baking—especially the breads and sugar—has caused Sally to gain over twenty-five pounds in the last seven years. She has had prediabetes and high cholesterol for the last two years. Despite my suggestions, she doesn't want to start on any medicine. "Doc, heart disease doesn't run in my family. Cancer does. And I stay on top of my screenings. Honestly, I'm not worried about my heart. I never have chest pain." Sally is focused on her cancer screening—and that is critically important. But the fact that heart disease doesn't run in her family doesn't protect her. She still needs to manage her risk.

When it comes to developing your personal program to prevent heart disease, it's important to understand what puts you at increased risk.

## Risk Factors

What are the risk factors?

**Age.** Just like with most other diseases, the risk of heart disease increases as we get older. For men, it starts to increase in the mid-forties; for women, it's a decade later, in the mid-fifties. But heart disease and heart attacks can occur at any age. I do want to point out that although it's rare, people in their thirties and forties can have heart attacks. When they do, there is usually a family history of heart disease.

**Family history**. As I noted earlier, there is a genetic component to heart disease. Some types (e.g., familial hypercholesterolemia) carry a greater predisposition than others. Genetic factors also play a role in high blood pressure and diabetes, which in turn increase your risk of a heart attack. It gets a little confusing at times, since it is also likely that people with a family history of heart disease share common environments and other factors that may increase their risk, such as smoking or eating a diet high in fat and sugar. We are doing much better in helping to determine the genetic mutations that might cause heart attacks, but we still have a long way to go in developing a simple blood or saliva test to determine genetic risk for most types of heart disease.

When we talk about family history, the age at diagnosis and family relationship matters. If your mother didn't have heart disease until she was eighty, that doesn't count as a family history when assessing risk. Rather, family history applies in calculating your risk if a father, brother, or son had heart disease before age fifty-five or a mother, sister, or daughter had heart disease before sixty-five. Some physicians and heart groups now suggest we should change that guideline to an increased risk if anyone in your immediate family had heart disease before age fifty. Premature coronary artery disease in a sibling can increase your risk by 40 percent. If your parent had heart disease at an early age, your risk increases by 60-75 percent. Therefore, it's important to find out what age family members were when they first had a heart attack or heart disease.

Another important aspect of learning your family history is that a positive family history of early heart disease is an indication that you may have a genetic tendency to develop high blood pressure or high cholesterol. That may require more frequent testing and monitoring.

Those are the risk factors you can't change. Let's focus on those you have control over.

**Obesity.** Excess weight puts additional stress on your heart, damaging the muscle and making it more difficult to pump blood throughout the body. Fat—particularly around the abdomen—releases hormones that can disrupt your metabolism, especially as it relates to blood sugar, blood pressure, and cholesterol. Fat around your middle becomes increasingly concerning as waist circumference becomes larger than forty inches for men and greater than thirty-five inches for women. You don't need to be checking your weight every day, but you should check it every couple weeks and look at trends. I know there has been some controversy regarding body mass index (BMI) as it relates to classifying people as overweight or obese. It still is one of the best measures we have right now, and it's important you know what your BMI is.

## HEART DISEASE TRENDS IN AMERICA

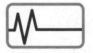

**LEADING CAUSE**
OF DEATH

**ONE PERSON DIES**
**EVERY MINUTE**
FROM CARDIOVASCULAR
DISEASE

**OVER 650,000**
**PEOPLE DIE**
EACH YEAR OF A
HEART ATTACK

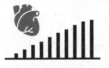

**MORE THAN 40% OF**
**AMERICANS**
WILL HAVE SOME FORM OF
HEART DISEASE **BY 2030**

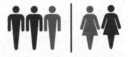

ESTIMATED THAT
**2 OUT OF 3 MEN AND**
**1 OUT OF 2 WOMEN**
WILL DEVELOP HEART DISEASE

**High blood pressure (hypertension).** Elevated blood pressure causes our blood vessels to narrow and get stiffer, often leading to dangerous blockages. This stiffness makes it harder for the heart to pump. In order to minimize this risk, your goal should be to keep your blood pressure around 120/80.

**Smoking.** The chemicals in smoke promote the creation of plaques, which stop blood flow throughout your body. Harmful substances in the smoke also make your blood thicker and more likely to clot. People who smoke often mistakenly think it makes them more relaxed, but in reality, chronic smoking increases your heart rate and blood pressure. Recent data suggests a fatal heart attack may often be the *first* sign of heart disease in middle-aged smokers. Vaping is also a risk factor. Studies suggest people who vape are more than 50 percent more likely to have a heart attack than those who don't vape. Sometimes patients mistakenly believe that vaping is safer—it's not!

**Physical inactivity.** As they say, "Sitting is the new smoking." Being a couch potato may increase your risk for heart disease as much as smoking. Not only does it increase obesity and diabetes; it speeds up premature aging, especially since it decreases your muscle strength. You've probably noticed that when you are deconditioned, it seems harder for you to breathe or you get tired more easily. That's partly because if you are inactive, it's more difficult to maximize oxygen consumption. All of this makes it much harder for your heart to function properly. Remember—your heart is a muscular organ, and you need to work to make it stronger.

**Diabetes.** Problems with keeping your blood sugar in a normal range can cause problems for your heart. Diabetes damages your blood vessels as well as the nerves that control how well your heart functions—how fast it beats and how well it pumps. Your heart must work harder when you have diabetes. Heart disease is pretty uncommon in women less than sixty years of age—unless you have diabetes! In general, you should strive to keep your hemoglobin A1c (HbA1c) less than 5.6 percent or a fasting blood glucose less than 100 mg/dL.

**Poor diet.** Food is medicine. You will see that mindset

throughout the book. What you eat affects all the systems of your body. Choosing foods that are low in nutrients and high in unsaturated fats, sugar, and sodium causes plaques to develop in your heart that can cause a heart attack.

**Hyperlipidemia.** We think of high cholesterol when it comes to our heart health, but the correct term is *hyperlipidemia*, which is basically a fancy word for an increase in different types of cholesterol. Cholesterol is a type of substance that we need to fulfill many of our body's functions. It's a mistake to think all cholesterol is bad. We all need some cholesterol to live. However, too much of the wrong types can be problematic. If you have high types of cholesterol, such as low-density lipoprotein (LDL) and triglycerides (TGs), or low good cholesterol, high-density lipoprotein (HDL), you are at increased risk of a heart attack. As mentioned, high cholesterol causes plaque to develop in your arteries. This plaque sometimes completely closes off a blood vessel, or a clot tears off and stops blood flow farther down your circulatory system. Hyperlipidemia is discussed in more detail in the testing section.

**Low iron.** Iron has an important job in our bodies as a crucial part of the proteins that deliver oxygen to our tissues. When iron gets too low, particularly as you get older or because of bleeding or nutritional deficiencies, the heart must pump harder, which can make you more tired than usual, as well as cause shortness of breath. All of this puts stress on the body, leading to a higher risk of heart attacks and strokes.

**Rheumatoid arthritis.** This type of arthritis (not osteoarthritis) not only destroys your joints; it also can destroy your blood vessels and your heart. The inflammation that exists in rheumatoid arthritis promotes plaque development. The presence of rheumatoid arthritis is an emerging risk factor that many doctors still aren't aware of, so it's important you know about it!

**Chronic kidney disease.** When your kidneys don't work properly, your heart often doesn't work properly either. Kidney disease can lead to low oxygen in the blood, which makes it harder for your body to perform its functions well. The kidneys also play a big role in blood pressure control, which, if not managed well, creates a shear force in your heart vessels. If your body is not eliminating toxins well, it can weaken your heart. Poorly functioning kidneys can also change the quantities of important electrolytes like calcium, potassium, and magnesium, which your body needs to maximize your heart health. Guess what the main cause of death is in patients with chronic kidney disease? Heart disease!

**Liver disease.** There's a condition called nonalcoholic fatty liver disease, which has two types: (1) simple fatty liver and (2) nonalcoholic steatohepatitis (NASH). Simple fatty liver, as the name implies, means you have fat in your liver, but you may not have any inflammation in your liver or damage to your liver cells. It usually doesn't get worse or cause liver problems. NASH is much more serious than a simple fatty liver. NASH means you have inflammation in your liver that can cause scarring and liver damage. This inflammation and the effect it has in elevating bad cholesterol and worsening insulin resistance all contribute to elevating your risk of heart disease.

**Gum disease.** The bacteria in your mouth, typically from your gums, often gets into your blood and can lead to plaque buildup in your arteries. Think of it this way: Plaque on your teeth can cause plaque in your heart. It's a bit more complicated than that, however, because there is also an increase in inflammatory cytokines when you have gum disease, which can increase your risk of developing heart disease. The bottom line: yes, you need to brush twice daily and floss!

**Asthma.** Your chances of having a heart attack go up about 70 percent if you have this lung disease. Even if you use an inhaler to keep it under control, your risk is still higher than normal. Because of your asthma, you also may tend to ignore chest tightness, which can be an early sign of a heart attack. Doctors don't know if breathing problems trigger heart attacks or if they simply have a common cause: inflammation.

**Medications.** Taking certain medications to treat other health conditions can increase your risk of heart disease. For instance, it's well known that certain drugs to treat cancer can damage heart muscle while helping you fight cancer, but did you know that ADHD medications also can have an impact, typically because of their effect on heart rate and blood pressure? In addition, if you use NSAIDs (e.g., ibuprofen) every day, that could potentially increase your risk due to their effect on sodium and water retention, as well as their impact on the flexibility of your blood vessels. It's always a good idea to check in at least every year with your doctor and pharmacist to weigh the risk and benefits of any medications you are on.

**Insomnia.** Over time, poor sleep can lead to unhealthy habits that can hurt your heart, including higher stress levels, less motivation to be physically active, and unhealthy food choices. There is a debate as to whether insomnia causes heart disease or heart disease causes insomnia. It's probably a bit of both. It is interesting to note that normally around bedtime and during sleep, your blood pressure and heart rate naturally decrease. If you aren't sleeping well, your blood pressure and heart rate stay up, which makes your heart work harder. Poor sleep also promotes inflammation, which can make plaques form more easily. If you have insomnia from obstructive sleep apnea, the potential mechanism for heart damage is a bit different. It changes the amount of pressure in different areas of the heart and results in an output that is not as strong. Low oxygen as well as frequent arousals increase resistance in your blood vessels.

**Migraines.** The risk to your heart appears to be strongest in the first year after diagnosis of migraine but persists for as long as two decades. During a migraine attack, blood vessels often constrict, reducing oxygen to vital organs— including your heart. Even though this is transient, repeated attacks can do long-term damage. There's also some belief that because people with migraines spend a lot of time lying down, it can make blood clots more likely. This is an emerging area of research, particularly in people who have migraine with aura, but it's important that you be aware of this potential increased risk.

**COVID-19.** Even though COVID-19 is a respiratory infection primarily affecting the lungs, it does increase your risk of heart damage. It does this primarily by preventing oxygen from getting to the heart. It also can cause inflammation of the heart, which disrupts your heart rate and rhythm, influencing how well it pumps. In addition, when the heart works harder to fight an infection, it may increase the risk of a heart attack.

**HIV.** If you are living with HIV, you have a greater risk of suffering a heart attack or heart failure than people without HIV. We used to think it was related to the antiviral treatments used to manage HIV, but the increased risk still persists with the newer treatments.

**Flu.** Your risk of having a heart attack increases if you also catch the flu. We are still learning the exact mechanism, but influenza can make your platelets more sticky, and that increases the risk of a clot. Getting a flu shot every year is an important way to protect your heart.

**Sex.** You may have heard that sexual activity has been linked to an increase in heart attack risk. But it's important to know that it is a very small one, especially if you're physically fit and in good health. For most people, sex can and should be an important—and healthy—part of life.

**Epilepsy.** Preliminary research has been showing a link between epilepsy and heart disease. It remains unclear whether it's due to seizures affecting heart rate and rhythm or if it is related to medications used to treat seizures.

**Menopause.** Women typically have protection from heart disease until they reach menopause, when they experience hormonal changes and changes in their lipid composition and weight (particularly the decrease in lean muscle mass). In addition, there can be an increased risk of heart disease based on certain medications used to treat some menopausal symptoms.

**Stress.** Mental health and physical health are connected. Leading a stressful life can increase your risk of heart disease. There was an interesting study published a few years back that looked at Twitter and found that tweets that showed negative emotions such as anger correlated with higher rates of heart disease deaths. Interestingly, the opposite was true as well—those who wrote tweets with positive emotions showed lower rates of deaths from heart disease. Of course, there are many more well-designed studies than just looking at tweets. More details about this in chapter 5.

**Depression.** As with stress, your mood affects how your heart and blood vessels function. Sadness can even reshape your heart, making it harder to pump blood to your brain and organs. I give more details about this in chapter 4.

**Loneliness.** Not only can social isolation and loneliness have a strong impact on your mental health, but they also increase your risk for heart disease. Data suggests that loneliness can increase blood pressure as well as reduce your immune function, which increases inflammation. This is especially true for women. It can increase risk up to 20 percent.

**Anxiety.** Recent data has shown that anxiety can lead to physiologic changes in your body that predispose you to heart disease. Men may be particularly affected by it, especially if they develop anxiety in middle age. I'll discuss this more in the chapters on depression as well as stress.

**Sudden or intense exertion.** Getting in shape will protect your heart in the long run, but doing too much could be dangerous. About 6 percent of heart attacks are triggered by extreme physical effort. The key is to listen to your body and not overdo it! For most people, the incremental risk of exercise causing a heart attack is minuscule.

**Eye disease.** We often say the "eyes are the window to the soul." They almost might tell you whether you are at increased risk for heart damage. A certain type of age-related macular degeneration may be a marker of disease elsewhere in your body. The particular type is called subretinal drusenoid-deposit phenotype, and a recent study revealed patients with this type of eye disease were ten times more likely to have heart disease compared to those who didn't have it. This is a good reminder to make sure you get a yearly eye exam.

**Gout.** If you frequently experience gout flare-ups, your risk of heart disease is increased. Since gout is partly a disease of inflammation with an increase in cytokines, it can temporarily increase your heart disease risk after a flare-up for up to four months afterward. Preventing gout flare-ups is important not just to preserve your joints but also to protect your heart.

**Cancer.** A cancer diagnosis increases risk of heart disease by 33 percent, particularly within the first year of diagnosis. This applies to all cancers. Some risk may be related to the treatments, but the diagnosis itself also contributes to increased risk. You can find more information about reducing cancer risk in my book *Take Control of Your Cancer Risk*.

**Cognitive impairment.** The mind and body are connected. It may be an issue of shared risks—meaning that if you have high blood pressure or diabetes, it increases your risk of dementia as well as your risk of heart disease. At the same time, when your mind starts to fail, often the rest of your body begins to have problems, including your heart. Given the increasing incidence of dementia, this will be an important risk factor to study further.

At this point you may be thinking, *What* doesn't *cause heart disease?* All of these factors assign a different amount of risk, and the more factors you have, the greater your risk. That's why it is so important to empower yourself with knowledge—to learn what you can and cannot control when it comes to your risk of heart attacks. The next few chapters tell you what you need to do!

## Summary

Knowing what causes risk is the first step in reducing it. Although genetic factors play a role, there are many other risk factors, most of which you can control. It's important to learn what puts you at risk and develop a strategy to help reduce that risk.

---

### ANSWERS

1. **False**. Genetics accounts for approximately 20 percent of heart disease.
2. **True**. Men can start to develop problems with their hearts in their forties; whereas women typically develop it a decade later.
3. **False**. What you eat plays a big role in your risk for heart disease, but it's the combination of risk factors and genetics that determines your total risk.
4. **True**. Although we often think of arthritis as merely painful joints, it's an inflammatory process that increases your risk of heart damage.
5. **True**. Healthy teeth translate to a healthy heart. The plaque that causes cavities and dental problems as well as inflammation can also cause problems in your blood vessels.

# CHAPTER THREE

# Estimating *Your* Risk for Heart Disease

## TRUE OR FALSE?

1. High cholesterol is the most important risk factor for heart disease.
2. C-reactive protein can help determine if you are likely to have a heart attack.
3. Current risk calculators give you an estimate of the risk of a heart attack in the next ten years.
4. Cardiac MRI is a useful study to look for plaques in your blood vessels.
5. You should get a stress test every five years once you're fifty.

*(Answers at end of chapter)*

GREG JUST TURNED FIFTY AND has a renewed focus on his health. He has done all the right cancer screenings, but he has struggled with his blood pressure and his cholesterol levels for years.

"I've got a stressful life, Doc" is his usual response when I talk to him about his blood pressure. "My blood sugar is good, so that's got to count for something," he quipped the other day to me. And it's true: normal blood sugar does help reduce risk—but doesn't eliminate it. Greg likes to look at numbers (he's an accountant!), so the other day I suggested we calculate his risk of having a heart attack in the next ten years. "You can do that?" he remarked in disbelief. I showed him the online calculator, we put the numbers in, and his score came back at 9.5 percent. "With that percent risk, we should talk about starting a statin" was my analysis, referring to a cholesterol-lowering drug. "That doesn't seem too high, does it?" Greg asked. Although people have different perceptions of risk, a 9.5 percent ten-year risk is considered moderately high and should be addressed through specific strategies to reduce it.

Based on genetics and lifestyle, everyone is at a different risk level for heart disease. How can you estimate *your* risk today as well as what your risk might be over the next few years?

The field of cardiology has done a great job of helping your doctor calculate your risk of a heart attack. But many doctors don't use these calculators, or they don't talk to you about them.

The American College of Cardiology along with the American Heart Association has an atherosclerotic cardiovascular disease (ASCVD) risk calculator that estimates your ten-year risk of having a heart attack or dying from heart disease. It's for people ages forty to seventy-nine, and it assumes you have not had a prior heart attack or stroke.

You need to input the following to calculate your score:

- Age
- Gender
- Race
- Blood pressure and whether you are treated for it
- Presence of diabetes
- Smoking status
- Total cholesterol and HDL cholesterol

Based on your results, you'll fit in one of four categories:

1. Low risk: You have less than a 5 percent chance of having a heart attack in the next ten years.
2. Borderline risk: There is a 5 percent to 7.5 percent chance of having a heart attack in the next ten years.
3. Moderate risk: You have a 7.5 percent to 19.9 percent chance of having a heart attack in the next decade.
4. High risk: You have a 20 percent or more chance of having a heart attack in the next decade.

The Framingham Risk Score is another tool used to predict your risk of heart disease. It is based on information gained from the Framingham Heart Study, hence its name. It's very similar, but there are a few differences in what numbers you put into the calculator. It's for people ages thirty to seventy-four who have no history or symptoms of heart disease. It provides a ten-year as well as a thirty-year calculation. (For people older than sixty-five who live in Europe, there are also risk calculators called SCORE2 and SCORE2-OP.)

If your doctor hasn't measured your risk score, you

should ask to have it done. And consider doing it yourself. I use these risk calculators all the time—on myself, family members, friends, and patients. For many people, it's a wake-up call that they need to make some changes. For others, it's a reminder to continue healthy living strategies and possibly incorporate new ones. That's where this book comes in—to give you science-backed recommendations designed to decrease your risk.

Some controversy does exist around these calculators as they relate to race. These risk scores may give worse predictions for Black patients compared to white patients, even when their risk profiles are identical apart from race. It's something to keep in mind. I would not stop using these scores because of potential bias but would put them into the overall context of risk assessment.

You need to have the score calculated and redo it every year if your risk is low or moderate to make sure it doesn't change to high. Like Greg, some patients express surprise about moderate risk being categorized as 7.5 percent and above. Yet that's the cut-off point where we see that specific strategies are needed to reduce risk, such as starting a statin (more on that in chapter 9).

That's one step to estimate risk. There are several other ways to help measure your risk of heart disease.

**Lab tests.** We often use lab tests to help diagnose disease. When it come to your heart health, labs can provide important information as it relates to risk. What do you need? How often? What's considered normal? I've got the answers for you.

**Lipid panel.** This is the test that tells you the levels of your different types of cholesterol. It's important to look at the different types, not just total cholesterol. These include:

- Total cholesterol
- LDL, the "bad" cholesterol
- HDL, the "good" cholesterol
- Triglycerides, the most common type of fat in your body

Each type is important to look at in your overall assessment.

For total cholesterol (includes both LDL and HDL):

- 200 milligrams per deciliter (mg/dL) or less is normal.
- 201 to 240 mg/dL is borderline.
- More than 240 mg/dL is high.

Sometimes people just ask about their cholesterol. That's a mistake, since it doesn't give you a complete picture of your risk. You need to focus on all aspects of your lipid panel, including HDL and LDL as well as TGs.

For HDL ("good" cholesterol), more is better. HDL is good because it helps pick up excess cholesterol and takes it back to the liver.

- 60 mg/dL or higher is good.
- 40 to 59 mg/dL is okay (men at least 40; women at least 50).
- Less than 40 mg/dL is low, raising your chance of heart disease.

For LDL ("bad" cholesterol), lower is better. It's bad because it builds up in artery walls, making them hard and narrow.

- Less than 100 mg/dL is ideal.
- 100 to 129 mg/dL can be good, depending on your health.
- 130 to 159 mg/dL is borderline high.
- 160 to 189 mg/dL is high.
- 190 mg/dL or more is very high.

For triglycerides, lower is better:

- Less than 150 mg/dL is normal.
- 150 to 199 mg/dL is considered borderline high.
- 200 to 499 mg/dL is high.
- 500 mg/dL and above is very high.

For those of you who find getting a lipid test a hassle, I have some good news. We used to think you needed to be fasting. That made it hard for some people to get this test, and they often didn't come back for it. Recent data suggests fasting is not required. If your triglycerides come back high, there is a chance you may need to repeat the test when you have fasted. But my recommendation is to get your lipids measured when it's convenient for you— whether or not you've been fasting. The American Heart Association recommends the test at least every four to six years starting at age twenty, as long as your overall risk of heart disease is low. If you already have heart disease or diabetes or have a family history of high cholesterol, you will need to get your cholesterol checked more often, possibly yearly.

Again, although we have normal ranges for each type, we need to take them all into account when determining risk and potential intervention. For example, if your HDL is high, that doesn't automatically balance out a high LDL. They all play a role and need to be measured.

**Lipoprotein (a).** Nowadays, we can do even more advanced testing of lipids; recognizing how many and how big the particles are makes a difference. Depending on your cholesterol levels and your underlying risks, your doctor might also measure lipoprotein (a), or Lp(a), which is a type of LDL cholesterol. Your Lp(a) level is determined by your genes and isn't generally affected by lifestyle, which helps assess your personal risk. It remains stable throughout life and therefore can provide useful information.

A high level is considered above 50 mg/dL.

If you have high levels of Lp(a), it may be a sign of increased risk of heart disease, though it's not clear how much risk. Sometimes to better quantify your personal risk, your doctor might order a Lp(a) test if you already have heart disease but you have normal cholesterol levels.

Not every doctor measures it, although the National Lipid Association does recommend testing for elevated lipoprotein levels if someone has a family history of early heart attacks—particularly before age fifty-five in men and sixty-five in women—or if LDL is greater than 190. Of note, doctors in Europe and Canada suggest everyone get tested once.

Again, a one-time baseline measure is usually all you need.

For completeness, there is apolipoprotein B (apoB). ApoB transfers cholesterol and triglycerides from where they are made to your different body tissues, which can then use them to produce energy as well as synthesize hormones. ApoB levels measuring above 110 mg/dL are considered high. Be aware that thyroid and kidney disease can falsely elevate it.

We are starting to see this measured more often. The European Society of Cardiology recommends measuring it to help assess heart risk, and the American College of Cardiology and American Heart Association recommend measuring it as part of a risk assessment enhancer for individuals with intermediate ASCVD risk. Some cardiologists also choose to monitor apoB after the start of lipid-lowering treatment.

**High-sensitivity or ultra-sensitivity C-reactive protein.** C-reactive protein (CRP) is a protein the liver makes as part of the body's response to injury or infection, which causes inflammation inside the body. Later in the book, I further talk about the role of inflammation as a cause of heart disease. If we could measure inflammation, that might give us a sense of risk. It seems like C-reactive protein may give us such information—or at least provide more data to create a better risk profile for you.

Typically, your doctor orders it when other labs or scores might suggest a moderate risk of coronary artery disease. High-sensitivity CRP (hs-CRP) tests may help quantify the risk further so you and your doctor can decide the next steps in your personal prevention program. Higher hs-CRP levels are associated with a higher risk of heart attack, stroke, and cardiovascular disease, perhaps up to three times the risk.

Because CRP levels can be temporarily increased by many situations, such as a cold, severe allergies, intense exercise, or going for a long run, the test should be done twice, two weeks apart. An hs-CRP level above 3.0 milligrams per liter (mg/L) indicates a higher risk of heart disease.

**Homocysteine.** Homocysteine is a common amino acid in your blood. You get it mostly from eating meat. Sometimes your doctor will measure it if you have a deficiency in vitamins $B_{12}$ or $B_6$ or folic acid. They might also measure it when assessing your heart risk, since high levels of it have been linked to early development of heart disease. If it's too high, it may damage the lining of your blood vessels as well as cause clots to form. An ideal level is less than 15 umol/L.

**Vitamin D.** Everyone seems interested in their vitamin D level. And yes, vitamin D can play an important role in overall health, especially as we talk about bone strength and immune function. When it comes to your heart, some preliminary data suggests low vitamin D could raise blood pressure, and that can elevate your risk of heart damage. It's reasonable to get it checked as part of your overall health assessment, but please don't start taking vitamin D supplements unless advised by your doctor. A normal range is between 20 and 50 ng/mL.

**Troponin T.** If you've ever been evaluated for a heart attack, you've probably heard the slang for troponin—or what ER doctors call "trops." We typically do this test in the setting of an acute heart attack. Measuring troponin T using a high-sensitivity troponin T test helps doctors diagnose a heart attack and determine the risk of heart disease. An increased level of troponin T has also been linked with a higher risk of heart disease in people who have no symptoms. It is important to note that it is *not* measured as part of a routine prevention strategy.

Besides lab tests, there are other diagnostic tests that don't involve taking blood.

**Calcium scores.** Several patients in recent years have been asking me about coronary calcium scores.

You've probably heard how good calcium is for your bones. There also is a relationship to your heart—but in the opposite way. You don't want calcium in your coronary vessels because the presence of calcium may mean you also have plaque.

By looking for calcium, your doctor might get an assessment of whether you already may have developed heart disease. I'm not talking about calcium that sometimes is measured as part of a blood test. To get a calcium score, a special CT scan checks for calcium by taking pictures of your blood vessels that carry blood away from your heart.

- A score of zero means no calcium is seen in the heart. It suggests a low chance of developing a heart attack in the future.
- A score of one hundred to three hundred means that moderate plaque deposits are possible. It's associated with a relatively high risk of a heart attack or other heart disease over the next three to five years.
- A score greater than three hundred is a sign of very high to severe disease and heart attack risk.

I've had it done. It takes only a few minutes. There's no injection of anything, and it doesn't hurt.

Again, this score doesn't look for plaque, so it's not 100 percent accurate. It looks for calcium and then correlates the amount of calcium to possible plaque. The coronary calcium scan isn't for everyone. During the test, your body is exposed to radiation—although it's a small amount.

Its role in risk assessment is still evolving. Typically, it's for people between the ages of forty and seventy who have an elevated risk (usually moderate) for heart disease but don't have symptoms, atypical symptoms, or a family history of early heart disease. It gives your doctor important information to determine if you need any additional tests or need to start any medicine, such as a statin.

**EKG.** You may have had an electrocardiogram—often called an EKG or ECG. They often are done before a surgical procedure (there's debate whether that should still be the case!). It's a test that records the electrical activity of your heart through small electrode patches that a technician attaches to the skin of your chest, arms, and legs. It's used to check for an abnormal heart rhythm as well as issues with blood flow, which could signal a heart attack. Sometimes it can also check for electrolyte abnormalities. It can also help tell if you're having a heart attack. The challenge is that as a tool for prevention, it provides little data for people at low risk who are asymptomatic. In fact, it may give you a false sense of security and deter you from getting other tests that can provide more of a complete risk profile.

If you are having *symptoms* of heart disease, such as chest pain, there are other types of tests to assess risk and help to determine if it's your heart that is causing the symptoms or perhaps another part of your body, such as your gastrointestinal tract.

**Stress Test.** There are different types of stress tests. We used to do them on everyone once they reached a certain age, but the accuracy isn't as good as we would like. Sometimes they are part of a life insurance physical or an executive physical. The goal is to see if there are any changes in blood flow with physical activity, which might mean you have heart damage.

The most common one is the *exercise stress test*. Sometimes people refer to it as a treadmill test. It lets your doctor know how your heart responds to being pushed. It essentially creates stress by having you walk on a treadmill or pedal a stationary bike. Your doctor is looking to see any changes in your EKG, blood pressure, and heart rate, as well as to see if any pain is reproduced.

**Pharmacologic or nuclear stress test.** This has different names, and you might hear it called a dobutamine, Persantine, or adenosine stress test. This is for people unable to exercise or when your doctor might need more details about your heart's blood flow than the typical treadmill test provides. You'll take a drug to make the heart respond as if you were exercising. This way, the doctor can still determine if there are blockages in the arteries. This is done by looking for areas of the heart that show good blood flow at rest and after "exercise."

**Stress echocardiogram.** An echocardiogram (often called "echo") is an ultrasound of the heart that shows its movement. A stress echo can accurately visualize the motion of the heart's walls and pumping action when the heart is stressed; it may reveal a lack of blood flow that isn't always apparent on other heart tests. This may demonstrate previous heart damage that could be impacting the blood vessels, valves, or even pumping strength. It can also check for any abnormal dilation of the aorta.

**Coronary angiogram or cardiac catheterization.** This is a procedure where a long, narrow tube called a catheter is inserted into a blood vessel in your arm or leg and is guided into your heart with the aid of a special X-ray machine. Doctors use contrast dye that they inject into your blood vessel through the catheter to create X-ray videos of your valves, coronary arteries, and heart chambers. This is not a general screening test for heart disease, but rather a "cath" (as it often referred to) is done to diagnose heart disease after other screening tests (that don't actually go into the heart vessels) when doctors need more information, or after a heart attack to see how well your heart is functioning.

As I mentioned, a cardiac cath is an invasive test. Although safe, there can be some risks, such as bleeding, allergic reactions to contrast dye, or damage to your arteries. Within recent years, there has been a push to develop tests that are "just as good" as cardiac angiograms but that don't require any tubes being put into blood vessels.

**Coronary computed tomography angiography (CTA).** This technique used a special CT scanner to look for blockages in the heart. A contrast dye is injected into your arm, and the CT scanner rotates, taking multiple highly detailed images of blood vessels and the heart. It typically takes just a few minutes. Since it's noninvasive, a coronary CTA can be performed much faster than a cardiac catheterization, with potentially less risk and discomfort to the patient, as well as less recovery time. If the results are abnormal, you may still need to undergo a "cath." CTA may be less accurate for some people, with a tendency to indicate more plaque than may actually exist, but they are continuing to get better, and they play an important role in evaluating your heart.

**Cardiac MRI.** Many people are familiar with an MRI with orthopedic and other procedures, but there are also some circumstances where we use it to get a good idea of how a heart is functioning. Unlike CT scans and X-rays, an MRI doesn't use any radiation. It uses powerful magnets and radio waves to make pictures of organs and structures inside your body. The technique collects data on your heart as it's beating and creates images throughout its pumping cycle. It's very good to see the structure of your heart, including the size and thickness of the four chambers and the valves, as well as how well blood is flowing through your major arteries. An MRI may be used in the setting of a heart attack or shortly afterward to see if your heart is healing. It is not typically used for screening for heart disease but may be done after other tests that require more information.

**PET scan.** A heart positron emission tomography (PET) scan is an imaging test that uses a radioactive substance called a tracer to look for disease or poor blood flow in the heart.

Unlike MRI and CT, which reveal the structure of blood flow to and from organs, a PET scan gives more information about how well your organs and tissues are functioning. A heart PET scan can detect whether areas of your heart muscle are receiving enough blood, if there is heart damage or scar tissue in the heart, or if there is a buildup of plaque in the heart muscle.

PET scans for heart disease are not widely available and definitely are not the first or second test ordered. Sometimes they can help determine if you need any specific treatments.

_____

## Summary

In order to develop your personal prevention program, you need to assess your risk. This can include lab tests as well as stress tests and imaging studies. Based on that information, you and your doctor can decide the best next steps. Keep in mind that this book is about primary prevention— preventing disease such as a heart attack before it occurs. The first step is diagnosis! Now that you know your risk, the next few chapters will tell you how to manage it.

## ANSWERS

1. **False**. Cholesterol is an important risk factor, but so are many others discussed in the previous chapter.
2. **True**. High-sensitivity C-reactive protein tests can provide useful information in helping to assess your risk of a heart attack.
3. **True**. Current risk calculators estimate your ten-year risk.
4. **False**. Although cardiac MRI can play a role in looking for plaques in your heart, it's not a tool used for general screening.
5. **False**. You should get a stress test when you have signs and symptoms of heart disease.

# CHAPTER FOUR

# Depression and Heart Disease

## TRUE OR FALSE?

1. Sadness can cause a heart attack.

2. Drugs to treat depression can cause a heart attack.

3. Experiencing grief is a normal part of life.

4. Approximately one of four people with heart disease suffers from depression.

5. Severe depression can physically break your heart.

*(Answers at end of chapter)*

MIKE AND RACHEL WERE MARRIED for thirty years. "We met while in college and have been together ever since" was a remark Rachel often made to friends. When Mike died suddenly of a heart attack, Rachel was heartbroken. "It felt like my life ended too" was her response. Even though she was in relatively good health—she was only about ten pounds overweight—Rachel herself died of a heart attack two years later.

We all have heard stories of someone who lost a spouse or child or close friend and died shortly thereafter. We wonder, *Were the deaths related?*

We used to think that depression and heart disease were two very distinct and different diseases—one related to mental health and one related to physical health. On the surface, depression and heart disease seem very different. After all, they are treated by two different specialties in medicine.

Upon closer examination, heart disease and depression have a few surprising things in common. They are the two most common causes of disability in the United States and other high-income countries. Both conditions cause significant harm to a person's overall quality of life.

But does depression cause heart disease, or is it a matter that if you have heart disease—a chronic condition—you can become depressed, just like you would with other chronic diseases like diabetes or arthritis? After all, no one *likes* going to the doctor all the time, concerned that their heart might stop beating! And when you're depressed, you often don't feel like exercising or focusing on what you eat. You may miss doctors' appointments or rely too much on alcohol and substances like tobacco. But does the pathophysiology of depression change the way your heart works, causing blockages?

A wealth of data over the last few years has changed our perspective about depression and the heart. We now know why depression is a significant risk factor for developing heart disease. Perhaps more importantly, we now know what heart-healthy steps you can follow if you or someone you know has struggled with depression.

## Depression and Your Heart

We've all been sad or lonely at times. Experiencing grief or occasionally feeling down is a normal part of life. But depression is much more than a temporary state of sadness. It's characterized by feelings of hopelessness, emptiness, and a loss of interest or pleasure in everyday activities. Depression can lead to anxiety, agitation, a loss of appetite, difficulty concentrating, and sleep disturbances, such as insomnia. Depression can last for months or years, and it can range from mild to severe.

In most cases, there is no one culprit that causes depression. As a few examples, it can be triggered by a combination of traumatic life events, your family history, and your relationship with drugs and substances. We know, for example, that depression can be caused or exacerbated by alcohol, prescription medications, and a variety of drugs of abuse. We also know that there is a strong genetic component to it: if you have family members who have grappled with depression, then you have an increased likelihood of experiencing it as well. Depression is multifactorial— biological, psychological, social, spiritual.

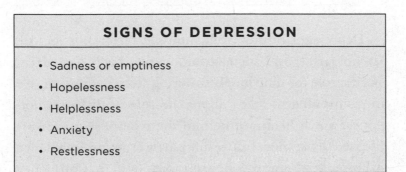

| SIGNS OF DEPRESSION |
| --- |
| • Sadness or emptiness |
| • Hopelessness |
| • Helplessness |
| • Anxiety |
| • Restlessness |

- Worthlessness. You may feel bad about yourself or your life or think a lot about losses or failures.
- Irritability. You may get more cranky than usual.
- Less interest in activities. Hobbies or games you usually enjoy may not appeal to you. You may have little or no desire to eat or have sex.
- Less energy. You may feel extremely tired or think more slowly. Daily routines and tasks may seem too hard to manage.
- Trouble concentrating. It could be tough to focus. Simple things like reading a newspaper, answering emails, or watching TV may be hard. You may have trouble remembering details. It might seem overwhelming to make a decision, whether it's big or small.
- Changes in the way you sleep. You may wake up too early or have trouble falling asleep. The opposite can also happen. You may sleep much longer than usual.
- Changes in appetite. You may overeat or not feel hungry. Depression often leads to weight gain or weight loss.
- Chronic pain. You may have frequent headaches, cramps, an upset stomach, or digestive problems.

Depression results from multiple factors: biological, psychological, and social components. Each can play a specific role for individuals suffering from depression. We are continuing to learn about the role of different hormones, which likely are behind the relationship to heart disease. Depression can result partly from an imbalance of hormones known as neurotransmitters that influence the brain. Two of the most important neurotransmitters that play a role in depression are serotonin and dopamine, the so-called "happy" or "feel-good" hormones. These hormones help to regulate your mood, emotions, and behavior. Serotonin influences your sleep-wake cycle, appetite, and metabolism, and it affects your ability to concentrate and think clearly. It also plays a role in the health of your heart. Dopamine has a wide range of important effects as well: it affects how you move and sleep and plays a crucial role in your motivation and ability to learn and stay alert. Like serotonin, it too can affect the health of your heart, influencing your heart rate, blood pressure, and blood flow.

Depression sometimes occurs when these hormones are not working properly or are released in the wrong amounts. Many studies show, for example, that having low serotonin—or in some cases having a lack of receptors in the brain that can respond to it—is a hallmark of depression. A deficiency in this happiness hormone or a lack of receptors for it in the brain can lead to anxiety, sadness, and despair—as well as insomnia, chronic pain, disordered eating, and trouble learning and concentrating. Chronically low levels of dopamine and norepinephrine can also be responsible for common symptoms of depression, such as fatigue, lethargy, a lack of motivation, and an inability to feel pleasure, known as anhedonia.

Studies in recent years have shown that when you have abnormal levels of these hormones, it can put your cardiovascular health in jeopardy. Remember how I said serotonin affects your heart? In a recent study published in the journal *Psychosomatic Medicine*, a team of researchers recruited a large group of healthy volunteers and examined their serotonin levels. Then they subjected them to a series of situations that made them sad, angry, or despondent and looked at how it impacted their heart health. They found that in the people who had the lowest levels of serotonin, the emotional situations activated cellular mechanisms that contribute to plaque formation and blockages, including a heightened immune response similar to what is seen in response to other factors like high cholesterol and smoking.

Among the changes the researchers saw was a spike in levels of inflammatory compounds, such as interleukin-1 and tumor necrosis factor alpha (TNF-α), which are known to cause a buildup of plaque in coronary arteries. The men and women who had normal levels of serotonin did not show these changes in response to the emotional situations. This demonstrates that serotonin does not just act on the brain; it also increases levels of inflammation, which raises the risk of heart disease.

It's not just the formation of blockages that can lead to a heart attack. Studies show that serotonin helps to regulate our heart rate and heart rhythm. It helps the heart pump better, plays a role in the constriction of our coronary arteries, and is involved in the formation of blood clots. Having too much or too little serotonin can cause these processes to go awry, which can contribute to the development of heart disease.

## Can Depression Break Your Heart?

One of the most striking examples of how depression and its accompanying hormonal imbalance strain the heart is a condition known as broken heart syndrome. This occurs when a person experiences profound grief and sadness. We see this, for example, in people who have lost a partner or a child. In fact, parents are at an increased risk for heart disease in the days after the death of a child, as well as years later. Your body releases a surge of stress hormones, such as adrenaline, that flood the heart, causing it to change shape and *literally* look like a broken heart. When this happens, the heart takes on the appearance of a pot with a round bottom and narrow neck.

## TAKOTSUBO SYNDROME

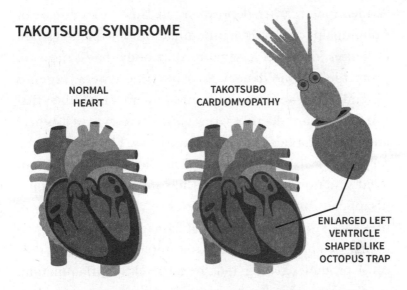

NORMAL
HEART

TAKOTSUBO
CARDIOMYOPATHY

ENLARGED LEFT
VENTRICLE
SHAPED LIKE
OCTOPUS TRAP

Broken heart syndrome was first described in Japan, where it was called "takotsubo cardiomyopathy" because the doctors who discovered it thought it caused the heart to resemble a *takotsubo*, a Japanese fishing pot that is used to trap octopuses. Broken heart syndrome is relatively rare, typically affecting only about 2 percent of all people who present with heart attacks. But its prevalence is rising, especially among older women. In a study published in the *Journal of the American Heart Association* in 2021, researchers found that broken heart syndrome was increasing at a rate six to ten times faster among women in the fifty to seventy-four age group than among any other age group.

In addition, the study found that roughly 90 percent of all cases occurred in women.

## Depression and Inflammation

As mentioned earlier, depression can cause heart disease by ramping up your levels of inflammation. The mental strain of depression sends a signal to your body that it needs to protect itself from danger. Your immune system responds by sending out an army of pro-inflammatory molecules that can fight off invaders like viruses and bacteria as well as heal and repair wounds and damaged tissues. These inflammatory chemicals are very helpful in the short term. In an ideal situation, they perform their jobs quickly and then disappear. But when you experience chronic depression, they stick around and do a lot of damage. They can perpetuate a vicious cycle in which the initial damage that they cause promotes greater and greater levels of inflammation.

Several studies have shown that depressed people have consistently higher levels of inflammatory markers, such as C-reactive protein, or CRP, a potent marker of inflammation that is associated with a higher risk of developing heart disease. One study that was published in the journal *Psychosomatic Medicine* in 2009 followed six thousand adults and found that depression as measured by the Beck Depression Inventory—a widely used instrument for detecting depression—was strongly linked to higher CRP levels. That's concerning because, as mentioned in chapter 3, high CRP levels can indicate elevated heart risk.

There are also many other inflammatory markers that skyrocket when people are depressed. In a large meta-analysis published in the journal *Brain, Behavior, and Immunity* in 2020, researchers analyzed 107 studies that compared immune function and inflammatory markers in 5,166 people with depression and 5,083 control subjects who did not have depression. They found significantly greater levels of inflammation in the depressed patients. In fact, many inflammatory markers were sharply elevated in the people with depression, including C-reactive protein, interleukin-3 (IL-3), interleukin-6 (IL-6), interleukin-12 (IL-12), interleukin-18 (IL-18), and TNF-α.

This study was by far the largest meta-analysis of immune markers in depression, and its findings were striking. TNF-α and the assortment of interleukins I just mentioned are known collectively as cytokines. These compounds are great at fighting off viral and bacterial invaders during an infection. But they can also cause a lot of collateral damage. When they flood your bloodstream for prolonged periods of time, they cause your blood vessels to constrict, increase your blood pressure levels, and promote blood clots that clog up your blood vessels. Studies show that TNF-α and other inflammatory cytokines cause plaques to form and rupture in your coronary arteries, triggering heart attacks and strokes.

## Endothelial Dysfunction

Another way that depression promotes heart disease is by causing something called endothelial dysfunction. The endothelium is a thin membrane that lines your heart and coronary arteries. It's made up of cells that help your heart vessels dilate and constrict. When the endothelium doesn't work properly, it impacts an artery's ability to dilate when it needs to—for example, during exercise. When the endothelium stops working properly, it can cause chest pain. It can also be an early sign of plaque and obstructions developing in your coronary arteries.

Many studies have indicated that depression triggers cardiovascular disease by causing endothelial dysfunction. For example, one study published in the journal *Circulation* found that periods of mental distress, which are typical of depression, can trigger endothelial dysfunction in otherwise healthy young adults. Another study published in *Circulation* also showed that psychological distress quickly causes the endothelium to stop working properly in healthy young adults. It concluded that endothelial dysfunction represents an important link between emotional stress and risk for heart disease. This study is particularly important, since it shows the effect of depression on the hearts of *young* people.

As if this weren't bad enough, depression causes destructive changes to your platelets as well. These are the blood cells that control blood clotting. Platelets can be lifesaving. When you have a wound, they rush to the site of your injury and clump together, forming a clot that prevents you from bleeding to death. But this can be deadly if your platelets form clots at the wrong place at the wrong time. When a plaque is disrupted or breaks off, platelets go to the site to "heal" the wall. This unfortunately can cause a blood clot, which obstructs blood flow, causing a heart attack.

A study published in *JAMA Psychiatry* over twenty years ago found that when platelets clump together in your arteries, they cause LDL cholesterol particles to cross into your arterial walls, creating plaque. This clumping together of platelets can also create arterial blockages, leading to heart attacks and strokes. A rather interesting study published in the journal *Biological Psychiatry* analyzed platelet activity in people with depression and in people without depression. It found that the depressed patients had abnormal platelet activation compared to the group of people who did not have depression, giving them what the researchers called an increased risk of stroke and heart attacks. The risk to your heart is quite real if you have depression.

## Heart Rate Variability

Depression can take a harmful toll on both your heart rate and your heart rhythm, which is another way that it causes cardiovascular disease. One new way that we can assess the health of your heart is by looking at something known as your heart rate variability (HRV). This is a measure of the variance in time between each beat of your heart. Many people have this feature as part of their wearables (e.g., Fitbit, Apple Watch, Oura Ring). Many people assume that their heart beats at evenly spaced intervals—for example, that it beats exactly once per second if you have a heart rate of sixty beats per minute. But if you're a healthy person, that's not the case: your heart might beat once per second, then speed up and beat again in less than one second, then slow down and take slightly longer than a second to beat again, and so on. This is because your heart rate is controlled by your sympathetic and parasympathetic nervous systems, which have opposing effects. Your sympathetic nervous system controls your fight-or-flight response, which tells your heart to beat faster, while your parasympathetic nervous system tries to keep your body in a state of calm, which slows your heart rate down.

In a healthy person, the push and pull between these two branches of the nervous system causes fluctuations in the time between heartbeats, which we call a high degree of heart rate variability. It may sound bad, but this is good because it indicates that your body is adaptable and can respond appropriately to both branches of the nervous system depending on what is needed at that moment. But when one branch of the nervous system routinely domi- nates, there is less variability between heartbeats, which we refer to as low heart rate variability. This is a common sign of poor cardiac function. Studies have found that heart rate variability tends to be significantly decreased in people with severe coronary artery disease or heart failure. A study published in the *American Journal of Cardiology* followed 808 people with heart disease for two and a half years and found that heart rate variability was a strong predictor of mortality. People with the lowest heart rate variability were five times more likely to die during the study than people with the highest heart rate variability. Go ahead and check your smartwatch or ring to see what your HRV is!

What's the link to depression? Studies have found that low heart rate variability is common among people who have depression. It occurs because depression causes reduced parasympathetic tone—or in other words, the sympathetic branch of the nervous system becomes more dominant. This means that it constantly sends stress signals to their bodies, pushing their hearts to beat faster than they should. This creates low heart rate variability, which puts an unhealthy strain on the heart.

The disruptive effect of depression on the heart plays

out in another way as well: it can cause abnormal changes in your heart rhythm. As I mentioned earlier, depression can drive inflammation. It is also associated with underlying hormonal changes like elevated levels of cortisol and thyroxine. These common features of depression can provoke a chronic condition known as atrial fibrillation, which causes abnormal heart rhythms. This can increase risk for heart attacks. In one study that was published in the *Journal of the American Heart Association* in 2019, scientists followed more than 6,600 people over a thirteen-year period after they were screened for clinical depression. They found that people who scored the highest on the depression screening test had more than a 30 percent greater chance of developing atrial fibrillation compared to people with test scores that did not indicate depression. A review of more than 500,000 people in over twenty-two studies measured baseline mood and depression symptoms and then followed participants for a year. People who had depression had an increased risk for both fatal and nonfatal heart disease.

––––––––––

## Chicken or the Egg?

Clearly, the relationship exists between depression and your risk for heart disease. But which comes first? Well, it's complicated. We know from large epidemiological studies that depression often precedes heart disease for many people. A meta-analysis of eleven studies published in the *International Journal of Geriatric Psychiatry* in 2007 found that people who experienced major depression had a roughly 64 percent higher risk of developing heart disease compared to people who did not have a history of depression. Another meta-analysis of twenty-one studies published in the *European Heart Journal* analyzed data on thousands of people and found that those experiencing major depression had an 80 percent higher likelihood of dying from coronary heart disease compared to people who did not struggle with depression.

While any history of depression increases a person's risk of developing heart disease, a study published in the *American Journal of Psychiatry* found that the more severe one's depression, the higher their likelihood of having heart disease. In one study published in *JAMA Psychiatry* in 2020, researchers followed roughly 146,000 people in twenty-one economically diverse countries (ranging from low- to high-income countries) for fifteen years. They found a 20 percent increase in cardiovascular events and deaths among people who reported four or more depressive symptoms during the study period. The risk of dying from cardiovascular disease increased progressively with the number of symptoms people reported, with the highest risk being in people with seven or more symptoms of depression. It seems that depression causes the same increase in heart disease and stroke risk as eating a poor diet. That's an important perspective for you to consider.

At the same time, having heart disease can make one depressed. It can change one's life, especially in the short term. Depressed persons often go to the doctor less, take their medications less frequently, experience poor sleep, and don't focus as much on a healthy lifestyle.

My point in telling you all this—and I did spend a lot of time on studies—is for you to realize that being depressed can increase your risk of a heart attack. As part of your personalized heart disease prevention program, you need to recognize the signs of depression and develop a strategy to treat it.

## Diagnosis Is the First Step

Everybody feels a little down now and then. Again, occasional sadness is a normal part of life. Most of the time it lasts just a few days and goes away on its own. As I mentioned at the beginning of the chapter, depression is different. It gets in the way of your daily life and makes it harder to do your typical activities. Don't assume "it will just go away" or that you can "snap out of it."

Because depression often goes undiagnosed, the key is to recognize the symptoms, especially early on, and talk to your doctor right away. I'm a big proponent of screenings. Doctors use different ones in clinical practice. A simple, quick one that I often use is called the Patient Health Questionnaire, or PHQ. There's a nine-question version as well as a two-question version. You don't have to wait for a doctor or therapist to administer it. You can do it for yourself or a loved one and bring the results to your health-care provider or mental health expert.

### DEPRESSION DIAGNOSIS

OVER THE *LAST TWO WEEKS*, how often have you been bothered by the following problems?

- Not at all = 0
- Several days = +1
- More than half the days = +2
- Nearly every day = +3

1. Little interest or pleasure in doing things
   - ❏  0
   - ❏  +1

❏  +2

❏  +3

2. Feeling down, depressed, or hopeless

❏  0

❏  +1

❏  +2

❏  +3

The PHQ score is obtained by adding the score for each question (total points). A score for this PHQ ranges from zero to six. If the score is three or greater, major depressive disorder is likely.

If you or a loved one screens positive, you should be further evaluated by a health professional.

---

## Lifestyle Changes That Can Help Relieve Depression and Protect Your Heart

Whether or not you have depression or struggle with occasional sadness, it's important to recognize the role of lifestyle.

Some of these tips can both help reduce your risk of depression and help as part of a comprehensive treatment strategy if you do have it.

**Avoid alcohol, smoking, and recreational drugs.** While these substances might seem like good stress relievers, they can trigger or exacerbate depression. Research by the National Institute on Alcohol Abuse and Alcoholism has found that heavy drinkers are four times more likely to develop depression than people who have never been heavy drinkers. Smoking and recreational drugs have also been shown to increase the likelihood that a person will develop depression. I also want to point out that although marijuana usage has become more widespread for both recreational and medicinal purposes, there is data that shows marijuana use can make depression worse or can even lead to depression.

**Give yoga a try.** If the thought of twisting your body into a pretzel makes you wince, consider the impact yoga has on your mind and body. We've known for centuries the positive benefit of yoga on mental and physical health, and we are seeing studies proving it. For example, in a systematic review published in the *Journal of Evidence-Based Complementary Alternative Medicine* in 2017, scientists analyzed data from twenty-three studies that looked at the impact of yoga on depression. They found that most studies showed that adopting a regular yoga routine for six weeks or longer helped to reduce symptoms of depression. It can help you re-center your thoughts and release powerful endorphins, those feel-good hormones that we discussed earlier involved in reducing pain and promoting happiness.

**Get a good laugh.** They say laughter is the best medicine, so it's no surprise that studies have shown that laughing frequently can change your mood. Who doesn't feel good at least for a little while after hearing a funny story or watching a comedy? Ever notice that when young kids get sad or mad, we make them laugh—and they feel better? Of course, it's more complicated for adults, but the act of laughing works by releasing serotonin and other feel-good hormones.

**Meditate.** Meditation helps people of all ages. In a recent meta-analysis published in the journal *Aging and Mental*

*Health,* researchers analyzed nineteen studies involving over one thousand seniors that looked at the relationship between meditation and depression. They found that assigning older people to practice meditation on a regular basis helped to improve their depression. Another meta-analysis and systematic review published in the journal *Frontiers in Psychology* in 2018 found that in teenagers and young adults under the age of twenty-five, adopting a mindfulness meditation routine helped to reduce symptoms of depression. Meditation takes practice. I always tell people you can't just go in a room, turn off the lights, and sit still. That's not meditation. Instead, consider some digital apps or try an online guided course. It's well worth your time, and there are many free ones available.

**Take time every week to do something you enjoy.** I know this is easier said than done, but it can be mentally and physically exhausting thinking about your health all the time. Make sure you find time to do things you like, whether or not it directly impacts your health. Just do it because you enjoy it. Maybe you like to play cards or listen to music. Gardening might be your source of joy. Maybe it's going out with a friend for coffee. The key is to spend some time every week on an activity that gives you joy. For this to work the best, consistency is key. You need to actively and purposefully plan it. Too often, we try to "fit in" things we enjoy. You must prioritize it and then protect that time.

**Get plenty of sleep at night.** Your sleep habits can have a substantial impact on your mood. That doesn't surprise you, does it? After all, how do you feel after a night of poor sleep? Imagine what the effect might be if you were to have chronic sleep issues. Many studies over the years have shown that people with insomnia are at much higher risk of developing depression. If you can cure the insomnia, you may be able to alleviate the depression. In a randomized controlled trial published in *JAMA Psychiatry* in 2022, researchers recruited 291 adults with insomnia and split them into two groups. One group was assigned to undergo two months of cognitive behavioral therapy to alleviate their insomnia, while the other group served as the control. After two months of treatment, the participants were followed for three years. The researchers found to their surprise that people whose insomnia went into "remission" were far less likely to develop depression. The study demonstrated that if you suffer from poor sleep habits, you can reduce your risk of developing depression by improving your sleep.

**Bathe in the forest.** I love the reaction from patients when I tell them to try a forest bath. Of course, it sounds like I'm telling them to literally bathe in the forest. But this type of bathing doesn't require taking any clothes off or carrying bug spray! Rather, forest bathing is spending some time outside in nature. You don't have to hike or play a sport. You simply go outside in a green area and let your senses go to work—smell, see, absorb what's around you. It doesn't need to be a forest. It can be a park, a garden, even a backyard. Numerous studies have shown that mood can improve with as little as twenty minutes a day, a few times a week.

**Start an exercise routine.** Exercise has powerful effects on the body and directly reduces your risk of heart disease. It also impacts your brain. It can boost your mood and help you fight depression. How do you feel after a run or a gym session? Like you are on top of the world. We even have a term called "runner's high," which is a feel-good sensation from running provided by the release of endorphins. Another reason for that great post-workout feeling is that exercise stimulates the release of brain-derived neurotrophic factor, or BDNF, a protein that stimulates the growth of new neurons and helps protect existing ones.

Studies show that depression is associated with atrophy in the central nervous system, specifically in a region of the brain called the hippocampus. According to research published in the *Proceedings of the National Academy of Sciences*, people with depression can lose up to 20 percent of the volume of their hippocampus, which explains many of the cognitive deficits and other symptoms seen in depression. But exercise can support the growth and maintenance of neurons in the hippocampus. According to a report from Harvard Medical School, this can improve nerve cell connections in the brain, which can help relieve depression. Be sure to check out the specific role of exercise in heart health, as well as a sample four-week routine in appendix A.

**Eat a heart-healthy diet.** As will be further discussed in chapter 6, what you eat plays a big role in your risk for heart disease. Food also plays a role in our emotional and mental health—think about how you feel after eating certain types of food. When you eat a piece of cake, you definitely feel differently than when you eat a salad—especially two hours later! There is a growing field of nutritional psychiatry that integrates food in an overall treatment plan. Dietary habits play an important role in both physical and mental health!

**Consider seeking therapy or medical assistance.** Depression often carries a negative stigma, which can prevent some people from seeking professional help. But you wouldn't avoid going to the doctor if you had diabetes, high blood pressure, or another chronic condition. You should look at depression just the same. While lifestyle changes can help to prevent or relieve the symptoms of depression, in many cases it may be necessary to get professional help as well. Therapy can often be enormously helpful, as can antidepressant medications. If you find that you've been struggling with depression and it's taking a toll on your quality of life, then I urge you to make an appointment with a doctor or a therapist.

## Can Medications for Depression Increase Risk for Heart Disease?

There are numerous medications to treat depression, and they work through different mechanisms. Every drug has risks and benefits, and they should be discussed with your doctor. For instance, some can cause weight gain, which can increase heart risk. The latest data on the newer medications (as opposed to older ones like the tricyclics) seem to have no direct effect in causing heart disease, especially if used for a short duration. There's even some emerging data on the potential benefit of certain antidepressants after one has had a heart attack.

## Summary

You need to recognize the role that depression can play in elevating heart risk. It is normal to occasionally feel sad as well as experience grief. If you are feeling down or depressed and it's bothering you most days of the week and preventing you from enjoying your usual activities, you should see a doctor or therapist. Treating your mood also treats your heart—the mind and body are connected!

| ANSWERS |
| --- |
| 1. **True**. Sadness, particularly prolonged sadness, causes physiological changes that increase your risk of a heart attack. |
| 2. **False**. Most medications, especially ones developed over the last ten years, do not directly increase risk of heart disease. |
| 3. **True**. Occasional sadness is a normal part of life. It's when it is prolonged that problems occur. |
| 4. **True**. Approximately 25 percent of people with heart disease suffer from depression. |
| 5. **True**. Although rare, severe depression can change the shape of the heart. |

# CHAPTER FIVE

# The Stress Factor

## TRUE OR FALSE?

1. Women experience more stress than men.
2. Ignoring stress can help it go away: "If you don't mind, it don't matter."
3. *Chronic* means that it's been going on for years.
4. A stressful work environment increases your risk of a heart attack.
5. Some stress is good. As long as it isn't daily, you don't need to change anything.

*(Answers at end of chapter)*

## ARE YOU STRESSED?

I bet you are—at least sometimes. I know that I get stressed occasionally.

We all have stress in one way or another, whether it's dealing with a job or relationship, caring for a child or parent, moving into a new house, or studying for an exam. It's how we manage it that is important when it comes to our risk for heart damage. In this chapter, I am going to discuss how stress and heart disease go hand in hand and provide some stress busters to help you manage it.

If you feel like you are more stressed nowadays than a few years ago, you are not alone. Since 2007, the American Psychological Association (APA) has been surveying thousands of Americans annually to track their stress levels. They found that people are increasingly stressed about work, relationships, their finances, family life, health-care, and other aspects of their daily lives.

In recent years, Americans have also reported increasing amounts of stress related to societal concerns like the opioid epidemic, mass shootings, and climate change. This was dramatically compounded in 2020 as the world grappled with the novel coronavirus pandemic. The APA found that the pandemic was a significant source of stress for 80 percent of adults, which took a physical and emotional toll on many people. The economy as well as geopolitics are creating additional stress.

As a result, many people are still suffering. About one in five adults said their heightened stress levels caused them to experience mood swings and increased feelings of tension. A similar percentage of people said they were prone to "snapping," getting angry very quickly, or screaming at loved ones.

What exactly do we mean by stress? When we talk about stress, it's important to answer this question: Have you experienced headaches, diarrhea, a racing heart, shortness of breath, difficulty sleeping, or neck tightness for a period of time?

Guess what? These are all symptoms that could mean you are under a ton of stress.

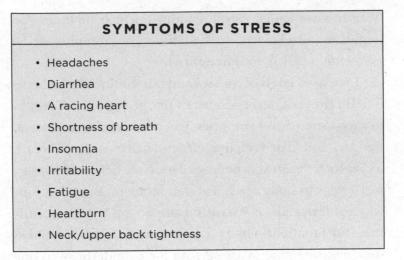

**SYMPTOMS OF STRESS**

- Headaches
- Diarrhea
- A racing heart
- Shortness of breath
- Insomnia
- Irritability
- Fatigue
- Heartburn
- Neck/upper back tightness

Stress is uncomfortable and makes you feel lousy. We have learned over the past two decades that stress can predispose you to heart disease and accelerate its progression. That's because stress triggers a cascade of physiological changes in your body that directly affect your heart and your blood vessels.

Let me explain.

## How Stress Affects Your Heart

When your body undergoes a stressful event of any kind, it activates a part of your brain—the hypothalamus—that regulates many of your hormones and bodily functions. It revs up your sympathetic nervous system, which controls your fight-or-flight response. As a result, your body starts pumping out cortisol, its primary stress hormone. But it's just not cortisol. It also secretes higher levels of a group of hormones called catecholamines, which includes epi-nephrine (also known as adrenaline) and norepinephrine (sometimes called noradrenaline).

Increased levels of cortisol and adrenaline can be bene-ficial in the short term—for example, giving you the energy to turn around and run when you sense you're in physical danger. You can feel the effect—heart racing, breath increasing, vision sharpening! These all help shift energy to where your body needs it at that moment. But when your cortisol levels are constantly ramped up by chronically stressful situations—like an overbearing boss who makes your job miserable or caregiving for an elderly loved one while also juggling parenting responsibilities—it can create an environment that damages your blood vessels.

It seems to make the cells of your circulatory system enter a state in which they almost go to sleep. It's like they stop functioning, which can result in plaque accumulat-ing in your blood vessels. Emerging data suggests that the higher a person's average cortisol levels, the greater the amount of plaque in their arteries.

Given that everyone does experience stress at some points in their lives, how do you know if stress is chronic? Although we don't have specific criteria around time, stress that lasts for several weeks or months is considered chronic.

What makes chronic stress so dangerous is that it leads to chronic inflammation. We know this from studying levels of different markers in blood. A study from just a couple years ago followed 350 people from mid-adolescence through adulthood and found that higher levels of stress were associated with increased levels of the inflammation marker CRP. As discussed in chapter 3, we often measure CRP to help us assess your risk of a heart attack, since inflammation prevents your blood vessels from functioning properly.

Another important reason stress can cause heart disease is that it spikes your blood pressure. The adrenaline and noradrenaline that your body pours into your bloodstream from stress cause your blood vessels to constrict or tighten up, which in turns makes your blood pressure climb. This can be a good thing if you need to act quickly to escape danger, and it definitely was helpful during our evolution. In our current environment, it can have dangerous effects. When your blood pressure is constantly elevated, it makes your arteries less elastic. This reduces the amount of blood and oxygen that can flow to your heart, which can lead to a type of chest pain called angina as well as heart failure. High blood pressure can also trigger strokes by damaging the arteries that provide blood and oxygen to your brain.

Chronic stress directly affects your personal risk for heart disease, but it also affects it indirectly by impacting blood sugar and other cell processes. It's a double whammy! A recent study of nearly one million adults found that diabetes was associated with an 18 percent increase in heart-related mortality, and the higher a person's average blood sugar levels, the higher their likelihood of dying from heart disease.

In *Take Control of Your Diabetes Risk*, I discuss the link between stress and diabetes. Stress causes high blood sugar, sometimes leading to the development of diabetes. Diabetes itself significantly increases your risk of heart disease in numerous ways:

1. Chronically high blood sugar levels can damage your arteries and the nerves that control your

heart. This can make it difficult for your heart to pump properly, depriving your cells of critical oxygen.

2. Over time, high blood sugar levels damage the endothelial cells that line the walls of your coronary arteries, making them more likely to form plaques.

3. High blood sugar can also fuel plaque formation by stimulating inflammation and causing disruptions in blood flow, known as shear stress, that injure the arteries.

4. High blood sugar levels reduce the amount of nitric oxide that your coronary arteries produce, causing them to narrow, which reduces blood flow to your heart.

———

## Your Environment and Stress

We know our personal lives cause us stress. But your professional life can as well. Your job could be hurting the health of your heart. Many large studies have shown that people who experience high levels of job strain are more likely to develop high blood pressure. The Coronary Artery Risk Development in Young Adults, or CARDIA, Study followed 3,200 healthy young adults for almost a decade to identify the habits and behaviors that are strongly linked to heart disease. The researchers found that people who experienced increasing levels of job strain were significantly more likely to go on to develop high blood pressure.

It doesn't matter what type of job you have, be it stocking shelves or managing money. The issue is: Do you feel busy and fulfilled at work or just busy and overly stressed? Studies have found that the worst kind of work environment for your heart is one that forces you to endure high demands and low control. People who feel that they have a significant workload but a low degree of control or decision making over their job are the most likely to experience health ramifications to their hearts. This is serious. Chronic stress related to impending deadlines at work has been linked to a sixfold increase in the risk of having a heart attack!

## Relationships: A Double-Edged Sword

It's also not entirely surprising that studies have demonstrated a strong link between heart disease and things like marital strain, bereavement, and social isolation. Relationships are a powerful source of social support. They can help protect you from the damaging physiological effects of stress. A lot of people have stressful lives. But if you have someone who cares about you to come home to at the end of the day, or a friend to call on the phone, or a family member to spend your weekends with, it can mitigate some of the chronic stress in your life. When you lack those lines of support, however, it can be yet another major source of stress.

One study of 325 adults published in the journal *Blood Pressure Monitoring* found that men and women who reported being in high-quality relationships with their spouses or significant others had lower blood pressure levels at home and at work compared to people who were in strained relationships or those who had no partner at all. Another study published in the *Archives of Internal Medicine* followed more than a hundred men and women for three years. It found that among people who reported "low" marital quality, the more time they spent around their spouses, the higher their blood pressure levels. But among people who reported "high" marital quality, spending more time around their spouses was associated with lower blood pressure levels. Relationships matter!

We also must recognize the role that caregiving plays in stress. Caregiving, especially for elderly or sick family members, is still mainly done by women. Caregivers focus on other people's health often at the expense of their own. In a recent study published in the *American Journal of Preventive Medicine*, scientists followed more than fifty-four thousand women across the United States for roughly four years. At the start of the study, none of the women had a history of heart disease or strokes. But by the end of the study, the researchers found that the women who had been overwhelmed by the stress of taking care of a sick spouse were significantly more likely to develop heart disease. Women who had spent at least nine hours a week caring for a sick or disabled loved one were nearly twice as likely to die from cardiovascular disease compared to other women.

## Acute Stressful Episodes vs. Chronic Stress

Although it's mostly chronic stress that causes problems, there are some instances where sudden and overwhelming stress can cause heart attacks. We have all heard the story of someone who got extremely angry, had a heart attack, and died. Studies have shown that episodes of anger or fear can cause an increase in the risk of heart attacks and strokes for several hours, days, or even weeks afterward.

This illustrates the impact our emotions can have on our health. Luckily, this type of catastrophic event is not common, but it does occur more often than we'd like. For instance, a study published in the *Journal of the American College of Cardiology* found up to a fivefold increase in the rate of death from cardiovascular disease among people living in Los Angeles shortly after the infamous 6.7 magnitude Northridge earthquake that struck there in 1994.

Another study showed that the rate of heart attacks in New Orleans roughly tripled in the three years after Hurricane Katrina. What was particularly surprising was that the stress of Hurricane Katrina had precipitated cardiac events in younger people too. Prior to Katrina, the average age among heart attack patients in New Orleans was sixty-two. But in the three years after Katrina, the average age of heart attack patients throughout the city dropped to fifty-nine. It may seem like only three years, but that's a big deal. The reality is that multiple factors are in play—the acute event, which is the sudden release of all those hormones that help keep you alive in the short-term, but also the associated chronic stress of loss of family and friends as well as one's home and job. The despair can be overwhelming for many people. This doesn't just impact our brains; it impacts our hearts—literally and figuratively.

Studies have also shown that even minor bouts of acute psychological stress can trigger cardiac events. For example, scientists looked at the impact of the 2016 presidential election on hospitalizations for cardiac events in a large health-care system in Southern California. They found that the rate of hospitalizations for heart attacks, strokes, and other cardiac events in the two days after the

2016 election were 1.62 times higher compared to the rate in the same two-day period one week earlier.

---

## Diagnosing Stress

I mentioned the symptoms of chronic stress, but honestly, they are not specific to stress—meaning, other conditions can present similarly. All too often, however, people who are stressed ignore it and think their symptoms are related to something else. This often leads people to not address it—or worse, they just consider it a natural part of life and something you "have to deal with."

Others are quick to recognize stress in others, but when it comes to themselves, they don't see it. Are you one of those people? You're sensitive to how other people are doing, but you don't show the same insights when it comes to yourself? I've got to tell you, it's quite a common phenomenon.

How do you know if you are stressed?

If you come to me as a patient, I ask this basic question: "Is your stress giving you an edge or getting in your way?"

If you answer that it's getting in your way, then we need to work on strategies to address it.

There are more detailed questions that I also use. There are a couple of different well-validated surveys that can be administered directly in a health professional's office, as well as great self-assessment tools you can do yourself to help you gauge the amount of stress in your life.

Because so much of stress is based on what you perceive as stressful, a good questionnaire is the Perceived Stress Scale. It asks about feelings and thoughts during the last month. It's only ten questions and focuses on how often you get upset, or feel you are unable to control important things, or feel angry or believe that things aren't going your way.

There's also the Perceived Stress Questionnaire. It consists of thirty questions and takes about fifteen to twenty minutes to complete. The scoring looks at your feelings of stress over the last year as well as over the last thirty days. It asks you to rate how often you feel rested, irritable, lonely, overtasked, frustrated, tense, judged, and mentally exhausted, as well as safe and lighthearted. What I like about the questionnaire is that it encourages you to think and assess how well you are doing. There's no right answer—and that's why we don't call it a test. Rather, it often is the first step in recognizing how much of an impact stress has on your mental health—and your physical health as well. Remember—there's no physical health without mental health!

These questionnaires should be done periodically. Once you and/or your doctor determine you are experiencing chronic stress, don't wait—take action. Remember, stress increases your risk of heart disease. It impacts the health of your blood vessels, the flow of your blood, and the amount of plaque you have. You cannot ignore it! Here are fifteen strategies to help you reduce stress in your life.

## Stress Busters

1. **Take a break from decisions.** Sometimes it can be exhausting having to make decisions all day. You can put your mind into overdrive by always having

to weigh options and decide a course of action. Many of those decisions can be weighty, and when you add them on to what's for dinner and what to do this weekend, you can reach a breaking point. It can be overwhelming. Instead, make some decisions into a routine—pasta every Sunday, walk every Wednesday, oatmeal for breakfast. This can help reduce the associated stress by eliminating the need to make a decision.

2. **Connect with others.** By this, I mean real connections! I'm not so much interested in how many "friends" you have on social media, but rather if you are connecting with family members, neighbors, and work colleagues. The COVID-19 pandemic made it much harder to maintain some connections, as well as make new ones. Virtual connection does play a role in our social lives, but in-person connection is also necessary at times. It is true that connecting with people can also bring upon stress, so first focus on those connections who have similar interests, hobbies, and perspectives. Spend time with people who bring you joy and positive feelings. Connecting with others often improves your mood and helps decrease your perceived stress. Keep in mind that building and maintaining friendships take time and work, especially as we all get older and have other priorities. I have a good friend who says he makes sure he sees friends for dinner or lunch at least twice a month. And he works on coordinating it—it doesn't just happen as we get older. Our interpersonal relationships are incredibly important as we work to reduce our personal risk for heart disease.

3. **Pet your dog or cat.** Anyone who has a pet knows they can be a great source of stress release. The human-pet connection is powerful and can improve your heart health by reducing stress. Science shows that when you pet a dog even for just a few minutes, your body releases feel-good brain chemicals like serotonin, prolactin, and oxytocin. At the same time, it decreases the amount of the damaging stress hormones that are released. That can mean lower blood pressure, reduced anxiety, and boosted immunity.

4. **Write out a to-do list, but don't put more than three things on it.** We often feel the stress from our mental to-do list. Do you ever find you are talking to yourself, reminding yourself of a bunch of things you need to get done? Too often, we do this at night, which makes it hard to sleep, or we do it in the morning, getting our day off to a stressful start. If you are prone to ruminating over things you need to do, writing them down can help take away some of the anxiety. But remember: keep the list short!

5. **Take time to recharge.** In our work and personal lives, we often put pressure on ourselves to be productive. You need time to decrease pressure. It's okay to feel lazy sometimes, and frankly you should make sure you feel lazy every week, even if it's only for an hour or two. Stop trying to be a superhuman—no one expects that. Every now and then, you need to just do nothing!

6. **Laugh.** Especially laugh out loud. I bet that after a bout of laughing, you feel less stressed and in a better mood. Have you ever said after a stressful day or

event, "Well, at least we can laugh about it"? Every time you crack up, increased oxygen courses to your organs, blood flow increases, and stress evaporates. In fact, just thinking about having a good laugh is enough to lower your stress hormone levels.

7. **Sing.** Music can help eliminate stress—even if it's just for a few songs. Several studies have shown enjoying music lowers stress. Turn up the radio in the car— and better yet, start singing. No matter how out of tune you are, singing can make you feel happier. Choral members who were surveyed said singing put them in a better mood and made them feel less stressed. Singing can also be good for your breathing and posture.

8. **Curb the clutter.** I find that looking at a messy desk, closet, or bedroom makes me stressed. It definitely brings on anxiety when you can't find the TV remote, an important paper, your iPad, or a book. So declutter to de-stress. Tackle one drawer, shelf, or tabletop at a time. An uncluttered space can feel satisfying and restorative.

9. **Practice gratitude.** Find something to appreciate in each important area of your life, such as your family, friends, work, and health. That perspective can help you get through tough times. Every week, try writing down three things you are grateful for but also why you are grateful for them. Forcing yourself to write them down will make you think about them, and that can help alleviate stress. There are various gratitude journals you can order to help you stay on track. We have learned from functional MRI and PET scans that practicing gratitude can help you rewire your

brain—turning off those areas that are associated with hyperarousal, anxiety, and stress.

## GRATITUDE POSITIVELY IMPACTS AREAS OF THE BRAIN

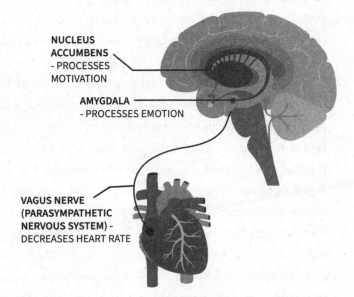

NUCLEUS ACCUMBENS - PROCESSES MOTIVATION

AMYGDALA - PROCESSES EMOTION

VAGUS NERVE (PARASYMPATHETIC NERVOUS SYSTEM) - DECREASES HEART RATE

10. **Set boundaries.** It's okay to say no to things that you don't really want or need to do. If you find yourself saying yes to a lot of things you'd rather not be doing, it might be time to start setting better boundaries. Boundary setting plays an important role in helping you and others understand what you can and cannot do. In many ways, it's about transparency—being transparent with yourself and others. Be sure to ask yourself, *Is it worth it to say yes?* If you can develop a framework to help you assess activities, that can help reduce your stress. Realistically, you will be putting more emphasis on your needs and feelings than those of others—but

hey, that can be a good thing to do! You can be assertive without being aggressive.

11. **Try mindfulness.** Mindfulness is a tool that I have learned to use over the past few years, and it does help me reduce stress and my perception of stress. People often feel more relaxed after some deep breathing and guided imagery. I do recommend that if you are new to mindfulness—which many people are—try some apps or directed instruction. Just like exercise, you need to practice meditation and use proper "form" to get the benefits.

12. **Get a massage.** Hand and foot massage can help release tension and the stress associated with it. You don't need to spend a lot of money. You can do it yourself with some lotion and knead your hand and feet muscles for five minutes. There are even some balls you can use on the bottoms of your feet, as well as back rollers for the neck. If you have never tried massage, you need to add it today to your stress-reduction strategies.

13. **Be kind to yourself.** Do you expect too much from yourself? We need to learn to be kind to ourselves. We treat others with compassion—and we also need to show self-compassion. Release yourself from self-criticism. Too often we traumatize ourselves with our own unrealistic demands to succeed. We end up becoming our own sources of stress. Combat this by being on the lookout for those overly critical thoughts, and slowly replace them with thoughts of encouragement. *I know I'm doing the best I can.* Now is the time in our lives for self-care.

14. **Get moving.** Being active is one of the best ways to reduce stress. I discuss this in detail in chapter 7.

15. **Seek professional help.** If your stress is making it difficult for you to function in your personal and professional life, you may need to seek help from a mental health professional. It's okay to admit you are not okay. You should consider scheduling an appointment to see if you are okay managing on your own or need additional help. Nowadays there are many ways, including telehealth, to get care quickly.

All of these strategies won't work for everyone, but surely you can find at least a few that you can incorporate into your life. It's time to recognize that stress affects not just your mental and emotional health but your physical health too. If you want to reduce your heart disease risk, you need to reduce your chronic stress.

Box breathing is a deep-breathing technique that can help you slow down your breathing. It works by distracting your mind as you count to four, calming your nervous system and decreasing stress in your body.

---

### HOW TO DO BOX BREATHING

- **Step 1:** Breathe in, counting to four slowly. Feel the air enter your lungs.
- **Step 2:** Hold your breath for four seconds. Try to avoid inhaling or exhaling for these four seconds.
- **Step 3:** Slowly exhale through your mouth for four seconds.
- **Step 4:** Repeat steps 1 to 3 until you feel re-centered.

---

## Summary

You can't ignore the role chronic stress has on the health of your heart. Even if you eat a healthy diet and exercise several days a week, if you suffer from chronic stress and don't address it, you are still putting yourself at increased risk for heart disease. Don't dismiss the signs of chronic stress.

| ANSWERS |
| --- |
| 1. **True.** Women do typically experience more stress than men. Men also suffer from stress and need to recognize the signs and symptoms. |
| 2. **False.** Ignoring stress is never a successful strategy in addressing it. It can make stress worse over time. |
| 3. **False.** Although chronic stress can go on for years, a few weeks of daily stress is considered "chronic" and needs to be addressed. |
| 4. **True.** The work environment is a common source of stress, which can damage your heart. |
| 5. **False.** Although it's the daily stress that adds up to heart damage, you need to be proactive in minimizing stress. Even repeated short episodes of intense stress can significantly increase your risk of a heart attack by decreasing blood flow. |

# CHAPTER SIX

## Diet Dictates Health

---

**TRUE OR FALSE?**

1. What you eat is more important than exercise in preventing heart attacks.
2. The quantity of calories determines your health.
3. Eating fat is okay as part of a heart-healthy diet.
4. Avoid dairy if you're trying to reduce your risk of a heart attack.
5. Reducing sodium is more important than reducing sugar when it comes to your heart.

*(Answers at end of chapter)*

---

THERESA HAS BEEN TRYING DIFFERENT diets off and on for the past fifteen years. "I started dieting after my first child was born. I've tried everything. And everything means paleo, vegetarian, keto, low carb, low fat. I lose weight for a couple months, and then I gain it all back. Sometimes, I end up weighing even more than before I started the diet. Heck, I even tried gluten-free, and I can eat gluten," Theresa often quips. "Tell me what to eat and I will do it."

Theresa is typical of many patients I see, as well as many friends. Eating healthy can be confusing. We all want to make the right food choices, but it's often not clear what we need to do. How often should we eat fish? Do we really have to consume fruit every day? Don't nuts have too much fat, or are they okay every now and then? Is coffee good or bad? And what about bread? This can all make your head spin.

The result: many of us don't eat a heart-healthy diet. Data from the 2019 Behavioral Risk Factor Surveillance System shows only 12.3 percent of adults consume the daily recommended amount of fruit, and only 10 percent consume the daily recommended amount of vegetables. Fewer than 20 percent of people eat fish one day a week; the rest eat none! I know people want to make healthy choices—they're just not sure what that means.

The first thing I tell people is that they fundamentally need to change how they think about food. You need to think, *Food is medicine.* Repeat that a few times. Heck, say it out loud! "Food is medicine." You need to realize that what you put in your mouth impacts all aspects of your body. What you eat is a critical component of your personal prevention program in reducing your risk of heart disease.

---

## Why Is Food So Important?

We know from volumes of research that what you eat plays a big role in your risk of heart disease. For example, thousands of studies have shown that your diet influences your blood pressure, heart rate, cholesterol and triglyceride levels, the amount of inflammation in your arteries, your blood sugar and insulin levels, and the amount of visceral fat that you carry around your waist and your internal organs—all of which have a major impact on your likelihood of developing heart disease. We all tend to know that to some degree, don't we? Think about it—how do you feel after you eat a bowl of ice cream versus a bowl of oatmeal? And how do you feel a couple hours later? You know it's having an impact on your body—and your weight. When we think of food as medicine, we also begin to recognize the significance of what we include as well as what we exclude. In many ways, what you eat is more important than how much you eat!

We've learned this because many more studies have shown us not only which foods and diets promote heart attacks and strokes but also which foods have the power to prevent them as well.

So, what should you eat?

Within the last few years, many doctor groups and experts have moved away from dictating calories and specific foods or recommending any specific diet. Rather, the focus has been on broad principles to follow. The goal is to keep it simple and provide a framework you can use *throughout* your life.

I really like what the American Heart Association did recently. In 2021, they convened a panel of the world's leading nutrition and cardiovascular experts to discuss the evidence behind food and heart disease. The result? A set of dietary guidelines that anyone can follow to optimize their cardiovascular health. It's exactly what I said you need—a simple and straightforward guide.

Here are the basic principles.

**Don't overconsume calories.** Too many calories can lead to weight gain, and weight gain can lead to heart disease. But even before we get to the number of calories you are eating, I want you to start thinking about the quality of the calories you are eating! The reason why this is so important is we used to think that all calories were created equal. We now have plenty of research that shows that that's not true. Let's be realistic—eating two hundred calories of broccoli is going to have a very different effect on your body than eating two hundred calories of candy. The broccoli will give you vitamins, antioxidants, and other nutrients that nourish your body. The candy will give you none of that. The broccoli will give you fiber that feeds your gut microbiome and helps to keep you full. The candy will make your blood sugar spike. Clearly, the calories in broccoli are better for you than the calories in candy, even when the portions have an identical number of calories.

When it comes to what you eat, the quality of the calories that you consume ultimately matters more than the quantity of the calories that you consume. But that does not mean that calories don't matter at all, especially when it comes to your weight. No matter what foods you eat, if you're consuming more calories than you burn, you will end up gaining weight—and carrying excess weight can increase your likelihood of developing heart disease. That's why it's important to exercise portion control. Large portion sizes, even for healthy foods, can contribute to positive energy balance and weight gain.

There are several factors that determine the number of calories you need to eat on a daily basis to avoid excess weight gain. These include your age, gender, height, weight, and physical activity levels. I'm not a big fan of counting calories, but I do think it's worthwhile to estimate your unique calorie needs as a reference point. That can help guide your general daily caloric requirements. There are several apps and websites that allow you to do this.

When it comes to calorie control, people often mistakenly believe that they need to cut a huge number of calories to gain benefit. And that often distracts people from the need for quality calories. The reality is that cutting just a small number of calories from your daily diet can have a big impact on your cardiovascular health. Consider a recent study in the *Lancet Diabetes and Endocrinology* that looked at what happened to a group of men and women who were asked to cut a modest number of calories from their diets and were then followed for two years. The participants were told that they could eat whatever foods they wanted, just as long as they ate less of them. The study involved 143 men and women, some of whom were overweight and some of whom were a healthy weight. On average, the participants reduced their calorie intake by 12 percent, or about three hundred calories a day, which is roughly the equivalent of a large bagel, one slice of pizza, or a medium serving of french fries at a fast-food restaurant.

## WHAT'S CONSIDERED A SERVING?

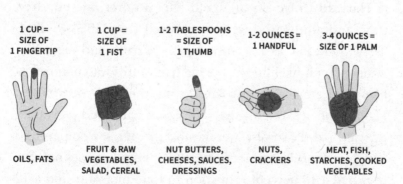

| 1 CUP = SIZE OF 1 FINGERTIP | 1 CUP = SIZE OF 1 FIST | 1-2 TABLESPOONS = SIZE OF 1 THUMB | 1-2 OUNCES = 1 HANDFUL | 3-4 OUNCES = SIZE OF 1 PALM |
|---|---|---|---|---|
| OILS, FATS | FRUIT & RAW VEGETABLES, SALAD, CEREAL | NUT BUTTERS, CHEESES, SAUCES, DRESSINGS | NUTS, CRACKERS | MEAT, FISH, STARCHES, COOKED VEGETABLES |

The researchers found that eliminating just three hundred calories a day caused sharp improvements in the participants' cholesterol and blood pressure levels. They had better blood sugar control and reductions in inflammation, and they lost weight and body fat. Yet a control group that did not make any changes to their caloric intake throughout the course of the study saw no improvements in their weight or metabolic markers.

We tend to think we need to make dramatic changes in our caloric consumption to gain heart benefits—and that can keep us from getting started or can cause frustration early on. Consider this instead, based on the data just discussed: Would you cut three hundred calories a day to improve your heart health and potentially extend your life span? Would you rather eat one hundred calories of food with powerful nutrients or mostly filled with sugar? That's how I want you to start thinking about food choices!

**Eat a wide variety of fruits and vegetables.** Mom was right: You should always eat your fruits and veggies. You should do it not only because your mom said so but also because many studies show that people who eat plenty of fruits and veggies live longer and have less cardiovascular disease. In a study published in the journal *Circulation* in 2021, scientists at Harvard University analyzed data on over one hundred thousand adults who were monitored from 1984 to 2014. They found that as a person's intake of fruits and vegetables went up, their likelihood of dying from cardiovascular events like heart attacks and strokes during the study went down. People who ate roughly five servings of fruits and vegetables per day had the lowest overall mortality rates. Compared to people who ate just two servings of fruits and veggies per day, they had a 13 percent reduction in total mortality and a 12 percent reduction in mortality from cardiovascular disease. (They were also less likely to die from cancer or lung disease.)

The researchers found that most fruits and vegetables contributed to this effect, with the one exception being starchy vegetables, such as white potatoes. They also did not find any benefit from drinking fruit juice. That's not surprising since fruit juice contains very little fruit, yet lots of sugar. It's better to stick to eating whole fruits and vegetables and to emphasize spinach, broccoli, peppers, tomatoes, zucchini, asparagus, brussels sprouts, and all other non-starchy veggies.

I often hear from patients that when they buy fresh fruits and vegetables, they often go to waste when not eaten in time. That does happen; it's happened to me many times. The solution: buy frozen or canned. We tend to think it's only fresh food that gives heart benefits. That's wrong. Frozen and canned food can often be just as healthy. Some canned tomato, corn, beans, and carrot products provide higher amounts of antioxidants than their fresh counterparts as a result of the canning process, which harvests them at the peak time. The quality and quantity of frozen and canned fruits has improved in the past few years. They also can be cheaper, and they last longer without having to worry about spoilage. I suggest you rinse your canned vegetables off and choose fruits packed in their own juice. You can also check the label to make sure there's not much sodium and sugar content added.

**Eat whole grains.** Oatmeal, barley, brown rice, and other whole grains have something in common with fruits and vegetables. They are great for your heart, but only when you consume them in their original form with their fiber intact (meaning their starchy endosperm, germ, and bran). The reason is that whole grains contain a lot of heart-healthy nutrients. The fiber that they contain is good for your blood pressure and blood sugar control. It helps to reduce inflammation, and it feeds your gut microbiome. Whole grains are a rich source of vitamins and minerals. But many packaged foods nowadays contain *refined* grains, which are grains that have been stripped of their fiber and other nutrient-rich components. Without their natural fiber, these foods are easy to overconsume and are rapidly absorbed into the bloodstream, causing blood sugar and insulin to spike.

Bagels, pastries, pasta, white rice, white flour, and white bread are some of the most common offenders in the refined-grains category, and you want to reduce how much of them you consume. In a meta-analysis that was published in the *BMJ* in 2016, scientists analyzed results from forty-five studies that looked at the impact of consuming whole grains on heart health. They found that consuming three servings a day of whole-grain foods, such as two slices of whole-grain bread and one bowl of brown rice, lowered the risk of developing coronary heart disease by 19 percent and reduced the risk of having a stroke by 12 percent. Compare that to no benefit demonstrated from consuming white rice and other refined grains. In another study published in the *Journal of Nutrition* in 2021, researchers followed more than 3,100 people for eighteen years and compared the impact of eating refined grains versus whole grains on cardiovascular disease risk factors. They found that people who ate four or more servings of refined grains each day had larger increases in waist circumference, blood pressure, and blood sugar levels over time than people who ate at least three servings of whole grains each day. The people who mostly ate whole grains had larger increases in HDL cholesterol, and they had greater declines in their triglyceride levels as well, all of which leads to lower risk.

**Choose lean or plant-based sources of protein.** Protein is one of the most important macronutrients you can eat. Along with fiber, it helps maintain the feeling that you are full, preventing you from overeating and thereby helping contribute to weight loss in many people. It helps you build and maintain lean muscle, and it gives your body the ability to repair damaged cells and tissues—all amazing benefits to be part of your personal heart disease prevention program! But you need to choose sources of protein that are going to do all these things *and* protect your heart.

There are several ways you can do this. One key way that the AHA suggests and that I try is eating plant-based sources of protein. That includes any food that's a plant or that is largely derived from vegetables, grains, and other plants. Some of the best foods in this category are beans, lentils, legumes, and nuts. These foods are high in protein and they contain plenty of heart-healthy fiber. They're also low in saturated fat and cholesterol, particularly compared to red meat. In a large meta-analysis published in the journal *Advances in Nutrition* in 2019, scientists reviewed data from twenty-eight rigorous studies that looked at the relationship between diet and cardiometabolic disease in tens of thousands of adults. They found that people who had the highest intakes of legumes (such as beans, lentils, and peas) and dietary pulses (the edible seeds from a legume) had a roughly 10 percent reduction in the incidence of heart disease and hypertension and a 13 percent reduction in obesity. In another meta-analysis published in 2019 in the journal *Nutrition Reviews*, scientists looked at data from nineteen different studies on the relationship between nut consumption and cardiovascular disease. They found that people who consumed several servings of nuts each day had a 15 percent reduction in heart disease and a roughly 20 percent reduction in their risk of dying from a heart attack or stroke. I find this particularly noteworthy because too many people are afraid of eating nuts. As long as you keep it to a handful of unsalted nuts, you are making a healthy choice.

Your goal should be to include plenty of these foods in your diet. But keep in mind that you don't necessarily have to be a vegan or vegetarian. (FYI: a vegan is someone who excludes all animal products from their diet, while a vegetarian is someone who excludes meat, poultry, and seafood but still eats dairy and eggs.) You can eat animal sources of protein and still gain cardiovascular benefits. The key with your animal-product consumption is to minimize your intake of red and processed meats while prioritizing fish and seafood, low-fat dairy, and lean poultry. For some reason, I find people often forget that fish is a great source of protein! That doesn't mean you can never eat a hamburger, hot dog, or strip of bacon. It just means that these foods should only be consumed occasionally—not every day. They certainly should not be a staple in your daily diet.

Fish, on the other hand, should be a central part of your diet because it contains omega-3 fatty acids, which help to lower inflammation and triglycerides. Many studies have found that consuming fish at least two to three times a week helps protect against heart disease. In one meta-analysis published in the journal *Nutrients* in 2020, scientists analyzed data from forty different studies on fish consumption and chronic disease and found that people who consumed large amounts of fish had a roughly 10 percent reduction in the incidence of heart disease and a 15 percent reduction in death from cardiovascular disease. While much of this benefit comes directly from eating fish, some of it might also stem from what is known as the substitution effect—meaning that by eating fish, you're avoiding less-healthy forms of protein, such as red and processed meat. Red meat contains plenty of saturated fat, which raises cholesterol, while processed meats, such as ham, hot dogs, bacon, and sausages, are rich in saturated fat as well as salt and preservatives. The key here is to *replace* red and processed meats with fish or poultry, and that can help reduce your risk of dying from heart disease.

At this point you might be wondering, *What about eggs?* For decades it was widely believed that eggs were bad for the health of your heart, since eggs seem to contain high levels of dietary cholesterol. But today we know that your body's cholesterol levels are largely driven by your genetics, and that for most of us, the cholesterol that we eat has a relatively negligible impact on our blood cholesterol levels. Saturated fat has a much larger impact on your blood cholesterol levels. For heart disease prevention, don't fret about eggs. One study published in the *Journal of the American Medical Association (JAMA)* followed nearly four thousand men and women for fourteen years while tracking their health and their diets. It found that consuming an average of one egg per day was "unlikely to have substantial overall impact" on the risk of developing coronary heart disease in healthy men and women. In a meta-analysis published in the *Journal of the American College of Nutrition*, researchers analyzed data from seven studies of egg consumption and cardiovascular disease. They found no association between egg consumption and increased or decreased risk of heart disease. Ultimately, eating a handful of eggs each week is unlikely to have much impact on your heart health.

When it comes to dairy products, making a switch from high-fat dairy foods to low-fat dairy may be beneficial. That's because dairy foods contain many important nutrients, especially fermented dairy foods like yogurt and kefir, which can provide benefits for your gut microbiome. But high-fat dairy foods tend to contain a lot of cholesterol-raising saturated fat. One of the most powerful demonstrations of the potential benefits of switching from full-fat to low-fat dairy foods took place in Finland fifty years ago. Back then, Finnish health authorities were worried about the country's excessively high rate of heart disease. They launched a campaign to encourage Finnish citizens to make substantial dietary changes. This included getting people to lower their cholesterol levels by encouraging them to switch from eating full-fat dairy to low-fat dairy. A study published in the journal *Preventive Medicine* found that the Finnish health campaign was quite successful: from 1972 to 1992, the saturated fat content of the Finnish diet dropped from 21 percent of total calories to 16 percent of calories, and the total fat content of the diet dropped from 38 percent of calories to 34 percent. During the same period, deaths from coronary heart disease fell by 55 percent among Finnish men and 68 percent among Finnish women. Researchers attributed about three-quarters of this decline to sharp reductions in cholesterol and other cardiovascular risk factors that were largely influenced by what people were eating. See—you can enjoy your milk and yogurt in moderation. But choose low-fat varieties when you can.

**Say "oh yes!" to olive oil.** One of the best things you can do for your cardiovascular health is to load up on olive oil and other rich sources of unsaturated fats. That's because studies have consistently shown that these foods can lower your LDL cholesterol levels *and* prevent heart attacks and strokes.

In an observational study of more than ninety thousand US health-care professionals, consuming even a small amount of olive oil was associated with reduced total mortality. Compared to men and women who rarely or never consumed olive oil (the lowest intake), those who consumed more than half a tablespoon (about seven grams) per day had a 19 percent lower mortality risk over a twenty-eight-year follow-up period, starting from an average age of fifty-six years.

Moreover, compared to those with the lowest olive oil intake, those with the highest intake had a 19 percent lower cardiovascular disease mortality, a 17 percent lower risk of dying from cancer, a 29 percent lower risk of dying from neurodegenerative disease, and an 18 percent lower risk of dying from respiratory disease during follow-up.

The researchers estimate that replacing ten grams per day of margarine, butter, mayonnaise, or dairy fat with the same amount of olive oil is associated with an 8 percent to 34 percent lower risk of death from various causes, including heart disease.

This study and others like it illustrate the remarkable cardioprotective effects of unsaturated fats. Two of the most important types of unsaturated fats are monounsaturated fats—which are found in avocados and olive and canola oils—and polyunsaturated fats—which are found in nuts, seeds, and vegetable oils, such as sunflower, corn, and soybean oils. You can also find polyunsaturated fats in fish and seafood. For optimal heart health, it's best that you minimize your intake of saturated fats like butter and replace them with unsaturated fats. That means that butter, despite how delicious it might be, should not be a staple in your diet. It's fine if you use some butter in the occasional recipe or use it on special occasions while baking. I'm not saying that you have to get rid of your butter in the refrigerator or any food that contains it. But for the most part, you should try cooking your foods in olive oil and canola oil instead of butter. Snack on nuts, seeds, and avocados. And try replacing the red and processed meats in your diet with fish and seafood so you get an extra dose of heart-healthy unsaturated fats.

**Beware of ultra-processed foods.** One reason the US and other countries have seen an explosion in heart disease, diabetes, and other diet-related diseases in recent years is because of what's happened to the food that we eat. A century ago, there was no such thing as an ultra-processed food. Now, ultra-processed foods make up *57 percent* of the calories in the average American's diet. That's according to a study published in the *American Journal of Clinical Nutrition* in 2021, which analyzed years of Centers for Disease Control and Prevention (CDC) data on what people eat. You've probably heard the term *ultra-processed food* before; it refers to packaged or fast foods that contain an array of additives, such as salt, sugar, industrial oils, sodium, artificial flavors, and preservatives. These are things like packaged cookies, donuts, pizza, pastries, ice cream, potato chips, white bread, and sugared beverages. Unfortunately, this ultra-processed dietary transformation that our country has undergone has been terrible for our health. Ultra-processed foods are engineered to have a long shelf life, but they are typically devoid of important nutrients like fiber, protein, and vitamins and minerals. They tend to spike blood sugar and insulin levels and stimulate a rise in hunger hormones and inflammation.

In a fascinating study published in the journal *Cell Metabolism* in 2019, scientists at the National Institutes of Health recruited a group of healthy adults and assigned them to live in a research facility for four weeks. During this time the researchers prepared all the participants' meals, tracked everything they ate, and closely monitored their weight, body fat, hormone levels, and other biomarkers. For one part of the study, the participants were assigned to eat a diet of mostly unprocessed foods. Then they were put on a diet of ultra-processed foods that contained similar amounts of calories, carbs, fat, and sugar. The participants were allowed to eat as much or as little of their meals as they wanted and they were allowed to have as many snacks as they wanted as well. At the end of the study, the scientists found that people were much hungrier when they ate the ultra-processed-food diet: they had higher levels of the hunger hormone ghrelin, and they ended up consuming an average of *five hundred extra calories per day*, which caused them to quickly gain weight.

It's a phenomenon we see duplicated time and time again in other studies. For example, researchers in 2021 followed over twenty-two thousand men and women for almost a decade and analyzed what they ate. They found that people who had the highest intakes of ultra-processed foods had a 58 percent higher risk of dying from cardiovascular disease and a 52 percent higher risk of death from a stroke. A similar study that was published in the *BMJ* in 2019 followed over one hundred thousand people for five years, and it too found that people who had high intakes of ultra-processed foods had significantly higher rates of cardiovascular and cerebrovascular disease.

What does all this tell you? It tells you that you need to put the book down and check your pantry, refrigerator, and freezer right now for ultra-processed foods. I hope you will get rid of them and not buy them again!

**Keep the amount of sodium in your diet to a minimum.** For optimal heart health, the American Heart Association recommends that you limit your sodium intake to no more 2,300 mg per day. That may seem like a lot, but most people consume much more. Before I get into more specifics, I want to clear up some confusion around salt versus sodium. According to the Food and Drug Administration (FDA), the terms *table salt* and *sodium* are often used interchangeably, but *they do not mean the same thing*. Table salt (also known by its chemical name sodium chloride) is a crystal-like compound that is abundant in nature. Sodium is a mineral and one of the chemical elements found in salt. Salt is what we add to our food when we use the salt shaker. We focus too much on the salt shaker when we need to focus on the sodium content. "I barely add salt to my food" is a common reply. I always tell them it's too much sodium that we need to worry about.

That's because according to federal dietary guidelines, the average person far exceeds the recommended limit and consumes roughly 3,400 mg of sodium per day. It's easy to overconsume sodium. That's because most of the sodium that we consume does not come from table salt that we add to our foods. Instead, it comes largely from processed foods like bread, pizza, potato chips, packaged snacks, cold cuts and cured meats, and fast-food meals. People who routinely consume a lot of sodium often have no idea unless they pay close attention to food labels. That's concerning because too much sodium can raise your blood pressure and heighten your risk of developing heart disease.

Consuming a lot of sodium causes your body to retain more water, and it makes it harder for your kidneys to remove fluid, which drives up the pressure in your arteries, making heart attacks and strokes more likely. Scientists have known about this relationship between sodium and blood pressure for decades. But studies in recent years have further illustrated the dangers of excess sodium consumption. In one study published in the *New England Journal of Medicine* in 2021, scientists recruited about eleven thousand adults and measured their daily sodium intake. Then, after following those people for an average of nine years, they looked at how a person's daily sodium intake affected their cardiovascular health. They found that people who had the highest sodium intakes, consuming up to 4,700 mg of sodium daily, had a 60 percent higher likelihood of having a heart attack or stroke than people who consumed the least sodium (an average intake of about 2,200 mg daily). Another study of fourteen thousand people published in *JAMA* found that people who had the highest sodium intake had an 89 percent higher likelihood of dying from a stroke and a 61 percent increase in the risk of dying from heart disease.

Cutting the excess sodium from your diet is a quick way to help reduce your risk of heart disease. Numerous studies have shown that steering clear of high-sodium foods can help protect your heart. In one study published in *JAMA*, researchers recruited thousands of adults and enrolled them in a lifestyle program to see how it would affect their blood pressure. They found that two changes had the greatest ability to lower the participants' blood pressure levels: losing weight and reducing their sodium intake. Each of these lifestyle changes caused significant drops in blood pressure, and we know high blood pressure increases risk of heart attacks.

Another study published in the *New England Journal of Medicine* in 2010 found that if Americans cut their daily sodium intake by 1,200 mg per day—in other words, reducing their sodium intake by about a third—it could prevent up to sixty-six thousand strokes and ninety-nine thousand heart attacks a year! Everyone would benefit, the researchers concluded, but especially people who are in high-risk groups, such as African Americans and people with hypertension. The cardiovascular benefits of reduced salt intake are on par with the benefits of population-wide reductions in tobacco use, obesity, and cholesterol levels. The takeaway here is to start taking a look at your daily sodium intake.

Sometimes I suggest to patients that they consider using a food tracker app for a couple weeks to track the amount of sodium in their diet. Look at labels—better yet, compare labels. If a frozen food has 900 mg of sodium, you're going to want to pass on that. I bet as you start looking at sodium content, you will be surprised by what you find. Your heart will thank you as you begin to cut back.

## FOODS HIGH IN SODIUM

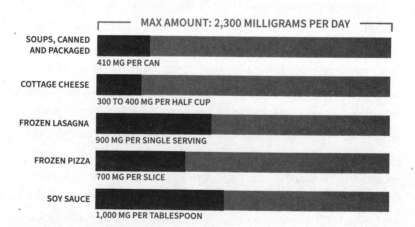

MAX AMOUNT: 2,300 MILLIGRAMS PER DAY

SOUPS, CANNED AND PACKAGED
410 MG PER CAN

COTTAGE CHEESE
300 TO 400 MG PER HALF CUP

FROZEN LASAGNA
900 MG PER SINGLE SERVING

FROZEN PIZZA
700 MG PER SLICE

SOY SAUCE
1,000 MG PER TABLESPOON

**Cut back on added sugars.** There's another little white crystal in your food that can be hazardous to the health of your heart. It's sugar, the other ubiquitous food additive that our tastebuds love but our arteries despise. The average American consumes a lot of sugar each day—about seventeen teaspoons' worth, according to the CDC. That's a lot more than the twelve teaspoons, or roughly 10 percent of an average person's daily calories, that the federal dietary guidelines recommend we limit ourselves to each day (and many experts think that allowing even twelve teaspoons is being too generous). Sugar is found naturally in some foods, like apples, oranges, and other fruits. But the sugar in fruit is not a problem because it comes packaged with plenty of fiber, vitamins, minerals, and other nutrients. And you can only eat so many apples or oranges in one sitting before you get full and step away from the table. The real problem is added sugars—the type of sugar that is isolated from plants and then added to foods in copious quantities. Large amounts of added sugars are one of the hallmarks of ultra-processed foods. It's not just the obvious foods like cookies, cakes, candy, and soda. Added sugars are found in everything from yogurt, ketchup, and breakfast bars to peanut butter, salad dressings, marinara sauce, and even bread. Bread always surprises people!

Ultra-processed foods tend to have a lot of added sugar and little or no fiber—the opposite of fruits and vegetables, which tend to have a lot of fiber and relatively small amounts of sugar. That's one reason ultra-processed foods are so bad for you. In a study published in *JAMA* in 2014, researchers followed tens of thousands of Americans for fifteen years and examined the relationship between their added-sugar intake and their cardiovascular health. They found that about 72 percent of adults got more than 10 percent of their daily calories from added sugar, and about 10 percent of adults got at least 25 percent of their daily calories from added sugar. That means that a whopping *one-quarter of all their daily calories* came from added sugar! The researchers found that people who went over the federal government's 10 percent daily-calorie limit on added sugars had a 30 percent higher risk of dying from heart disease, while those who got 25 percent or more of their daily calories from added sugar had triple the risk of dying from heart disease. One of the largest sources of added sugar in the American diet is sugary beverages, including soda, juice, sweetened teas, and energy drinks. These foods are particularly problematic. In a large meta-analysis published in the *International Journal of Clinical Practice* in 2016, researchers looked at food consumption and cardiovascular outcomes in over three hundred thousand adults and found that for every serving of sugar-sweetened beverages a person consumed on a daily basis, their risk of having a stroke climbed by 13 percent and their likelihood of having a heart attack rose by 22 percent. Overall, people who drank large amounts of sugary beverages had a 20 percent higher risk of having a heart attack compared to people who consumed few or no sugary beverages.

That's why it's a good idea to reduce the level of added sugar in your diet as much as possible. You can start by cutting out sugary beverages. If you routinely drink them, switch to water, unsweetened tea, sparkling water, or water flavored with lemon or lime. Because sugary drinks are such a concentrated source of added sugar, eliminating them from your diet will drastically reduce the amount of sugar you consume. Another step you can take is to cut back on fast foods and ultra-processed foods. These foods are a major source of added sugar in the American diet. By slashing your intake of sugary drinks, fast foods, and ultra-processed foods, it's very likely you'll be able to get your added sugar intake down to a more reasonable level.

## FOODS HIGH IN ADDED SUGARS

THE FDA RECOMMENDS ONLY 50 GRAMS PER DAY OF ADDED SUGARS BASED ON A 2,000 CALORIE DAILY DIET, WHICH IS 12.5 SUGAR PACKETS.

SUGAR ONE PACKET=4 GRAMS OF SUGAR

| Food | Sugar packets |
|---|---|
| HALF CUP OF PASTA SAUCE | 3 |
| HALF CUP OF GRANOLA | 3 |
| 8 OUNCES OF YOGURT | 8 |
| PACKET OF INSTANT OATMEAL | 3.5 |
| 2 TABLESPOONS OF SALAD DRESSING | 3 |
| CUP OF BREAKFAST CEREAL | 5 |
| BOTTLE OF TEA | 8 |
| CUP OF PACKAGED FRUITS | 10 |
| TABLESPOON OF KETCHUP | 1 |
| 8 OUNCES OF ENERGY DRINKS | 6.5 |
| BOX OF RAISINS | 6 |

**Consider your beverages.** What you drink is as important as what you eat. We tend to not focus on beverages when we think of food, but you need to as part of your personal heart disease prevention program.

When it comes to beverages, I always tell people the

change you could make today to improve your heart health would be to replace any soda (diet or regular), iced teas, lemonades, and juices with plain water. It can be a quick fix, and you will automatically decrease the number of daily calories you consume, as well as eliminate a lot of sugar. That's why above I pointed out the sugar content of beverages.

I know some people get concerned about coffee. Well, I have some good news to share! Coffee in moderation can be helpful to your heart—typically two to three cups a day. However, this doesn't include frappuccinos, cappuccinos, or mochaccinos!

In a recent study, researchers looked at 500,000 people over a ten-year period. They looked at varying levels of coffee consumption, ranging from up to a cup to more than six cups a day, and the relationship with heart rhythm problems (arrhythmias); cardiovascular disease, including coronary artery disease, heart failure, and stroke; and total and heart-related deaths among people both with and without cardiovascular disease. Patients were grouped by how much coffee they reported drinking each day: zero, less than one, one, two to three, four to five, and more than five cups per day.

In general, having two to three cups of coffee a day was associated with the greatest benefit, translating to a 10–15 percent lower risk of developing coronary heart disease, heart failure, or a heart rhythm problem, or dying for any reason. The risk of stroke or heart-related death was lowest among people who drank one cup of coffee a day. Researchers did observe what's called a U-shaped relationship with coffee intake and new heart rhythm problems. The maximum benefit was seen among people drinking two to three cups of coffee a day, with less benefit seen among those drinking more or less.

**When it comes to drinking alcohol, less is more.** Can you drink to your health? You've probably heard this saying before, perhaps while sitting around a dinner table and raising a glass in the air for a toast. It also seems to be a component of life in France and other areas of the Mediterranean world, where the incidence of heart disease seems to be much less. But when it comes to alcohol and your cardiovascular health, it's important to recognize that recent data suggests alcohol consumption should be limited as part of an overall wellness plan. That's largely because of the role it may play in increasing certain types of cancer. (I discuss this in more detail in my book *Take Control of Your Cancer Risk*.) In addition, the relationship between alcohol consumption and heart health follows what experts call a J-shaped curve. That means that a little alcohol may be good for you, but as your intake rises, the risk of disease rises sharply too. In small quantities, alcohol can dilate blood vessels, act as a blood thinner, and possibly raise your HDL cholesterol. But in large quantities, alcohol can be toxic to your liver and kidneys and constrict your blood vessels.

In one study published in the *Journal of the American College of Cardiology* in 2010, scientists followed 245,000 people for over a decade and looked at how their drinking habits affected their health and mortality. They found that people who were "light" drinkers—meaning they consumed one or fewer drinks per day—had a 31 percent reduction in their risk of dying from heart disease. People who were "moderate" drinkers, meaning they consumed two or fewer drinks per day, had a 38 percent reduction in their risk of dying from heart disease. But people who drank three or more drinks per day saw almost no benefit compared to the light and moderate drinkers. Those who abstained from drinking saw no benefit either.

In a meta-analysis and systematic review published in the journal *BMC Public Health* in 2020, another group of researchers analyzed data on alcohol intake and health from seven rigorous studies involving thousands of participants. They too found that light to moderate drinking had a slightly protective effect against cardiovascular disease. Light drinkers had a 32 percent reduction in the incidence of heart disease, and for moderate drinkers there was a 28 percent reduction in heart disease. There's some belief that people who drink small amounts of alcohol also exhibit healthy behaviors, which may account for the risk reduction. Just so you know—in most studies "moderate alcohol intake" means no more than two drinks a day for men and one drink a day for women—no more than five days of the week.

A recent analysis in the *Lancet* concluded that age also needs to be factored into alcohol consumption. For instance, the analysis suggests that for young adults aged fifteen to thirty-nine, there are no health benefits to drinking alcohol, only health risks, such as accidents. For adults over age forty, consuming a small amount of alcohol might provide some health benefit.

Bottom line: alcohol consumption is clearly a bit more complicated than we originally thought, especially as we look at heart health—but also overall health. Here's the takeaway: if you currently don't drink alcohol, don't start. Don't use it as a strategy to reduce your risk of a heart attack. And if you do drink alcohol, then limit your intake. Remember: less is more!

## Summary

There's a French phrase, *Dis-moi ce que tu manges; je te dirai ce que tu es*—Tell me what you eat, and I will tell you what you are. A more traditional American quote would be "You are what you eat." Whether we say it in English or French, it means the same: what you put in your mouth on a daily basis over many years plays a major role in whether you develop heart disease. To reduce that risk, you must develop a new perspective on food and use it as a tool to reduce your risk of heart disease. That means consuming more fruits and vegetables and whole grains, as well as substituting fish for red meat and low-fat dairy for full-fat dairy. You need to pay attention to the beverages you drink as well as how you cook your food. Finally, use snacking as a way to continue to eat healthy foods throughout the day.

### ANSWERS

1. **False**. Although the type of food you eat plays a critical role in determining your risk of heart disease, we can't say it is more important than exercise. Both are important.

2. **False**. The latest research suggests it's not just about the quantity of calories but also the quality.

3. **True**. Eating fat is okay as long as it is monounsaturated or polyunsaturated fats and is done in moderation.

4. **False**. Low-fat dairy (versus full-fat dairy) can play a role in reducing your risk of heart disease.

5. **False**. Reducing sodium and sugar are both important when it comes to your heart. It's difficult to say which is more important.

# CHAPTER SEVEN

# Exercise and Prevention

BILL IS FIFTY-FIVE YEARS OLD and has arthritis and prediabetes. He's been overweight, as he jokes, since he was born. "I've tried everything, Doc. I can try to work on what I eat, but I'm just too old to go to the gym. I'm active enough at work. I don't need to be muscular. Besides, with my arthritis, I get a lot of joint pain. Don't you have a pill or something I can take?"

Like many people, Bill doesn't like to exercise. He

doesn't see the connection between exercise and the benefit to his heart. He thinks it's a "nice to have" rather than a "must-have" as part of his personal heart disease prevention program. Sometimes as we get older, we view exercise as something that's just for our looks. As a result, it seems less important and less of a priority. That's unfortunate because exercise is essential to helping ward off heart attacks and strokes. When it comes to a magic pill, exercise is as close to it as we have.

Exercise has many benefits for your overall health, not just your heart. Exercise:

- Strengthens your bones, delaying or preventing osteoporosis.
- Increases muscle endurance and builds and maintains muscle mass.
- Promotes joint flexibility.
- Improves function of respiratory muscles and steadies one's breathing patterns.
- Releases endorphins, helping to reduce anxiety and depression.
- Decreases dangerous free radicals, helping with protection of the brain.
- Strengthens memory by improving neural activity and connections.
- Improves the quality of sleep, which we now know impacts both the length and quality of our lives.
- Enhances metabolism, helping keep your blood sugar and body weight under control.
- Generates loss of body fat, including around internal organs.
- Reduces chronic inflammation.

When it comes to your heart health, exercise packs a powerful punch, both directly and indirectly. It does this in several ways:

1. **Exercise makes your blood vessels more flexible and elastic, which improves blood flow and circulation.** It helps get oxygen to those parts of the body where it's needed, when it's needed. Exercise keeps our arteries from becoming hardened and full of plaque as we age. Part of the way it does this is by producing nitric oxide. Nitric oxide is a vasodilator. This means it makes the inner muscles of your blood vessels relax and widen, reducing the amount of stress placed on them. This causes an increase in blood flow and a reduction in your blood pressure. Think of it like a pipe in your bathroom: If it starts to get clogged with hair or other debris, the water doesn't flow well. If it gets backed up completely, it can burst. Your blood vessels basically work the same—they are essentially pipes. Exercise helps prevent them from getting clogged and keeps your blood pressure healthy. A recent analysis of more than sixty studies found that on average, people who start an exercise regimen can expect to see their systolic blood pressure fall by five points and their diastolic blood pressure decline by three points. These might seem like modest changes in blood pressure, but they can have dramatic consequences: a five-point drop in systolic blood pressure corresponds to a roughly 14 percent reduction in stroke mortality and a 9 percent reduction in heart disease mortality.

2. **Exercise helps your platelets work better.** Platelets are the small, disc-shaped fragments that circulate

in your blood. Platelets are something of a double-edged sword: When you're injured, they clump together and plug holes in your arteries to stop you from bleeding. But they can also form blood clots in your brain and coronary arteries, leading to heart attacks and strokes. Exercise makes your platelets less sticky, helping prevent them from causing unnecessary blood clots. This helps to reduce the stickiness of your blood, which lowers your risk of heart disease.

3. **Exercise helps keep your blood sugar under control.** It does this by making your muscles act like a sponge that soaks up excess glucose circulating in your bloodstream, lowering your blood sugar levels. A recent study found that exercise causes *a fivefold increase* in glucose uptake in your muscles and that this increase in glucose uptake lasts up to forty-eight hours after a single bout of exercise. Longer term, it makes your body much more efficient at using glucose. This is particularly important given the epidemic of diabetes and prediabetes. Exercise helps you overcome the resistance to insulin that is the hallmark of type 2 diabetes, making your cells more sensitive to insulin so glucose can get into your cells for the energy you need. Even a relatively short session of high-intensity exercise, lasting as little as twenty minutes, can cause improvements in how well insulin works for up to twenty-four hours. Better blood sugar control results in lower risk of heart disease!

4. **Exercise can reduce your cholesterol level.** Although your cholesterol level is influenced by genetics and

diet, exercise can help you manage it, especially if you lose weight. Exercise stimulates enzymes that help move LDL from the blood to the liver. From there, the cholesterol is converted into bile, which is either digested or excreted. So the more you exercise, the more LDL your body expels. What I find particularly important is that exercise increases the size of the protein particles that carry cholesterol through the blood. Some of those particles are small and dense; some are big and fluffy. It's the small ones that are dangerous because they squeeze in the linings of your blood vessels and cause damage. At the same time, exercise—particularly strength training—increases the amount of HDL, which can be protective.

A few years ago, researchers recruited over one hundred sedentary, overweight adults with high cholesterol levels and split them into four groups. Three of the groups were assigned to participate in one of three exercise programs, while the fourth group served as controls. One exercise group was instructed to do high amounts of high-intensity exercise. They did the caloric equivalent of jogging twenty miles per week at 65–80 percent of their peak oxygen consumption levels. A second group did low amounts of high-intensity exercise, the equivalent of jogging twelve miles per week. The last group did low amounts of moderate-intensity exercise, equivalent to walking twelve miles per week. After six months, the study found that each of the exercise groups had greater improvements in their cholesterol profiles than the control group. They saw substantial reductions in the concentrations of their LDL and small LDL particles. They also had increases in the average size of their LDL particles, sharp reductions in their triglyceride levels, and significant increases in their HDL cholesterol levels—which you now know are associated with better heart health.

5. **Exercise produces a hormone called irisin, which may help white fat cells transform into brown fat cells.** It does this by binding to certain receptors on fat tissue. This is important since white fat cells are responsible for storing fat and brown fat cells help burn fat, helping you to lose weight. This change in fat composition will make you less insulin resistant as well. Granted, most of these studies have been done in mice, but it's an exciting area of research.

These are just some of the benefits of exercise you may experience as part of your personal heart disease prevention program. I spend a lot of time talking to patients about what they should do. But lately, I also ask patients to consider what the impact of their *not* exercising could be. Doing it has numerous benefits, but what's the result of not being active?

I said earlier in the book that sitting is the new smoking. What I mean is that just as smoking is bad for your health, so is too much sitting. Having couch-potato tendencies is hazardous to your heart. Physical inactivity is the fourth leading risk factor for early death worldwide, contributing to more than three million deaths annually.

One large systematic review published in the *International Journal of Environmental Research and Public Health* followed 650,000 people around the globe and concluded that a lack of exercise leads to 6 percent of all coronary heart disease deaths worldwide. It also found that engaging in high levels of physical activity lowered the risk of coronary heart disease and stroke by up to 30 percent. That's because, as you just learned, exercise helps prevent diabetes, obesity, hypertension, high cholesterol, and high levels of inflammation—all of which promote heart disease. Exercise helps prevent premature death. Isn't that what we all are trying to do as part of any disease-prevention, healthy lifestyle program? Of course it is! As we now are beginning to realize, low cardiovascular fitness may be more dangerous than smoking.

By this point, I know what you're probably thinking. *Okay, Dr. Whyte, I'm sold. I know I need to exercise, but* how much *and* what type *should I actually do?* There are countless ways you can exercise—and figuring out which types and how much to do can be confusing. But it doesn't have to be.

Let's take a look.

## Exercise Guidelines: How Much Should You Do?

When it comes to exercise, it's about quantity and quality. The American Heart Association recommends the following when it comes to how much and how intense exercise should be when it comes to your heart:

- 150 minutes per week of moderate-intensity aerobic activity, or
- 75 minutes per week of vigorous aerobic activity, or
- a combination of both, preferably spread throughout the week.

Add moderate- to high-intensity muscle-strengthening activity (such as resistance or weights) on at least two days per week.

You are probably wondering what counts as "moderate." Moderate-intensity physical activity means your target heart rate should be 50 to 70 percent of your maximum heart rate. The maximum rate is based on a person's age. An estimate of a person's maximum heart rate can be calculated as 220 beats per minute (bpm) minus your age.

You can use your smartphone or other devices/apps to monitor your heart rate. Or you can go low tech and estimate your exercise intensity with the simple talk test. To perform the talk test, see if you can talk or sing while performing the activity. If you're doing moderate exercise, you should be able to talk, but not sing. If you're doing vigorous exercise, you shouldn't be able to say more than a few words.

There's also the Perceived Exertion scale, where basically intensity is determined by how you feel your heart rate and breathing. A one means it's very light exercise and a ten means it's very heavy. For most people, a three or four is moderate. Of course, this is subjective, but if you are consistent in using this scale, it does work.

Some of you may be thinking, *That's a lot of time to exercise every week!* At first, it does seem that way . . . but when you break it down and think of the benefits, it can be manageable. And remember, those are goals. For most people, it's going to take a while to reach them.

I suggest you try breaking your exercise up into increments of thirty or forty-five minutes on several days of the week, or even ten minutes several times a day. I often tell patients—and myself some days—everyone can do something for ten minutes! Try not to let more than two days per week go by without being active.

I like this approach because you don't want to have too many days in between times you exercise. If you do something every day, or every other day, it will keep you on track. If you're new to exercise and just getting started, it's okay to do whatever you can. Remember: doing something is better than doing nothing. As long as you are consistent and build up to 75–150 weekly minutes, you will reap a benefit.

For those of you who are limited in time, what should you focus on? Should you just do cardio, or is strength training more important? It's the classic cardio-versus-weights debate.

**Cardio vs. strength training . . . how do they compare?** Step into any gym in America, and there are usually at least two rooms. There's the weight room, with rows of dumbbells and exercise machines designed to make you stronger. And then there's the "cardio" room, with rows of treadmills, stationary bikes, and other machines designed for aerobic workouts. Most people prefer one type of workout to the other. But is one necessarily better for your heart than the other? I know cardio implies the heart—literally, it means *heart!*—but studies show that when it comes to doing cardio or strength training, the answer is you should do both. That's because each gives different benefits, and you'll get more bang for your buck by combining them. We didn't always realize this, and most people focused on cardio or aerobic activity, but recent studies have changed our thinking.

In 2020, researchers published a study that followed a half million Americans for almost a decade and looked at the types and amounts of exercise they did and how it affected their risk of dying from heart disease and other chronic conditions. The scientists found that people who did seventy-five minutes of weekly strength training had an 11 percent lower risk of dying from heart disease or cancer during the study period compared to people who did not meet the weekly strength training recommendations. Those who met the recommendations for weekly aerobic activity had a 29 percent lower risk of dying from heart disease compared to those who didn't do the recommended amount of aerobic exercise. But the people who did both strength training and aerobic exercise fared the best: their risk of an early death was reduced by an astounding *40 percent*. The study found that survival rates were especially good for people who did at least seventy-five minutes per week of "vigorous" physical activity. But it also showed enhanced survival for people who did 150 minutes per week of light to moderate physical activity.

Does this surprise you? There's more! In another study published in the *American Journal of Epidemiology* in 2018, researchers followed 80,000 adults for about fourteen years and looked at how exercise affected their health and mortality rates. They found that both strength training and aerobic exercise were great for overall health. People who did at least two sessions of strength training per week or who did at least 150 minutes of moderate-intensity aerobic activity lowered their likelihood of dying during the study by 16 to 23 percent. The study found that aerobic exercise was particularly good for cardiovascular health, lowering the likelihood of developing heart disease by 22 percent. But like many other studies of exercise, the study showed that doing both strength training and aerobic exercise each week provided the most bang for your buck. People who did both types of exercise had the lowest rates of heart disease and the highest survival rates overall: they slashed their odds of dying early by roughly 30 percent.

## SPECTRUM OF CARDIO AND STRENGTH EXERCISES

### ♥ CARDIO          💪 STRENGTH

**MODERATE**

| CARDIO | STRENGTH |
|---|---|
| BRISK WALKING | SQUATS |
| LIGHT JOGGING | BICEP CURLS |
| ELLIPTICAL MACHINE | MODIFIED PUSHUPS |
| SWIMMING | FOREARM PLANK |
| CLEANING HOUSE | RESISTANCE TRAINING |
| GARDENING | PILATES |
| DOUBLES TENNIS | YOGA |

**VIGOROUS**

| CARDIO | STRENGTH |
|---|---|
| RUNNING | BURPEES |
| STAIR CLIMBING | WEIGHTLIFTING |
| CYCLING | HANDSTANDS |
| SINGLES TENNIS | KETTLEBELLS |
| RACQUETBALL | MARTIAL ARTS |
| JUMP ROPE | SHOVELING SNOW |
| HIKING UPHILL | MOUNTAIN CLIMBING |

Sometimes women avoid strength training for fear of getting "bulky" or muscular. You need to recognize that strength training does *not* mean bodybuilding! Skipping strength training is a mistake when it comes to your heart. Researchers at Harvard University looked at exercise and deaths from heart disease among 29,000 women who were observed for twelve years. They found that doing aerobic exercise or moderate amounts of strength training protected women against cardiovascular disease and promoted longevity. But again, the most benefit came from doing both types of exercise. Women who did moderate amounts of strength training and at least 150 minutes per week of aerobic exercise had the lowest rates of death from heart disease.

---

## What About Machines or Free Weights?

Both can play an important role, especially when people are starting an exercise program. Free weights allow for a more natural range of motion and help teach your body to control weights, often involving the core. The challenge is that you do need to do the exercise correctly. And too often, we tend to think we can lift a lot more than we actually can, resulting in potential injuries with free weights. Machines can be very useful, especially as you are learning new exercises. They help teach the body certain movements and allow you to more easily estimate the weight you should use. The weight moves on a fixed path, which is not always the natural arc. I often suggest a mix, with more machines early on and then free weights as one becomes more advanced. Just know which things each type can do.

The data from studies is clear: to prevent heart disease and extend your life span, it's better to do a combination of aerobic exercise and strength training. But what about intensity? Does that matter?

For many people, increasing the intensity of your workouts can boost the cardiovascular benefits that you gain. Researchers followed about forty-five thousand men for over a decade and looked at the relationship between their exercise levels and their risk of developing coronary heart disease. After adjusting for age, weight, diet, cholesterol levels, and other variables, the researchers discovered that various types of physical activity lowered coronary heart disease risk. For example, men who ran for an hour or more each week had a 42 percent risk reduction compared with men who did not run. Training with weights for thirty minutes or more each week was linked to a 23 percent lower risk of heart disease. Rowing for an hour or more each week lowered heart disease risk by 18 percent. And doing a brisk walk for 30 minutes each day was also associated with an 18 percent reduction in risk.

What I found really exciting is that the researchers determined that doing any of these exercises at a high intensity was associated with the greatest risk reductions. The study showed that if two people did the same amount of exercise each week—whether it was one hour or five hours per week—the person who exercised at a higher intensity gained the greatest amount of cardiovascular protection. This was true for running, walking, rowing, swimming, weight training—you name it. Why am I telling you this? It's because I want you to take away this message: increasing the amount of exercise you do and upping the intensity of it from low to moderate or from moderate to high is among the most effective strategies for lowering your risk of heart disease. I love it when I hear that my patients are going on walks with their spouse or friends. But my advice is: don't make it just a social event—you gain more benefits by putting effort in and breaking a sweat.

The beauty of exercise is that even if you have been inactive for a very long time, starting an exercise program right now can still reap many benefits. In a study published in the journal *Circulation* in 2018, researchers recruited fifty-three middle-aged adults who were previously sedentary and split them into two groups. One was assigned to take part in a two-year high-intensity exercise program. The other group served as the controls. Those who took part in the exercise program did high-intensity aerobic exercises like running, cycling, and swimming as well as high-intensity workouts with weights. The control group did a combination of low-intensity workouts that involved things like yoga, stretching, and balance training. After two years, the researchers found that the high-intensity exercise group had much greater improvements in their cardiac function than the control group. They had substantial decreases in cardiac stiffness, for example, and larger increases in their maximal oxygen uptake—both of which indicate greater protection against heart failure and other cardiovascular diseases. The researchers concluded that regular bouts of high-intensity exercise could help reverse the cardiac effects of sedentary aging in middle age.

Wow! This is good news! Why? Say you haven't been exercising for a decade or even more. Research shows that even if you restart in your forties and fifties, you get almost the same protection from heart disease as people who have always exercised. At the same time, you can't live in the past. Just because you were active as a teenager and young adult doesn't mean you can be a couch potato now. The benefits of exercise to your heart come from consistency.

## Do I Really Have to Do Ten Thousand Steps?

Depending on your height and stride, ten thousand steps is about five miles a day. It's a good goal, but there's no real science to support it. For most people, six to seven thousand is helpful. It does vary by age. For example, data suggests 4,500 steps for women in their seventies can help them live longer, which includes protecting their heart. Focus on improving your daily step count over time.

---

## Ready to Start?

Let's be realistic. It's hard getting started, and it's hard being consistent. Over the years, I've heard it all—and frankly, I've used many of these excuses myself.

Barriers to exercise:

- I'm too old.
- I have no time.
- I don't want to get hurt.
- I don't like to sweat.
- I just got my hair done.
- I'm not dressed properly, and there's nowhere to change.
- It's too cold/hot.
- I don't know what to do.
- I need to get in shape before I can go to gym. (This one is my favorite!)

There are a couple of factors behind these feelings. First, there is a lack of understanding of the health benefits. You may not be aware of all that exercise does for your heart. It's exactly what my patient Bill was alluding to at the beginning of this chapter. Sometimes we equate it with how we want to look, but we really need to equate it with how we want to feel—and how long we want to live and the quality of that life. The second is the low priority that we put on incorporating exercise into our lives. Even when we know being physically active is valuable, we still have trouble getting started, and we place other priorities ahead of it.

We have become so accustomed to instant gratification in today's society that unless we see benefit right away from exercising—typically weight loss or bigger muscles—we lose interest. Exercise does have short-term benefits, but it's the long-term results from making exercise a part of your overall lifestyle that help you reap the most benefits for the heart. Yes, it can be delayed gratification given most heart benefits come later, but if you could prevent or delay a heart attack—and the sudden death or long-term disability that can be associated with it—wouldn't you want to?

I know people sometimes are a bit scared to get started. Most people can safely start to exercise. If you have been sedentary for quite some time, I do suggest, though, you see your physician before starting. It's also a good idea to see a doctor if you have high blood pressure, existing heart disease, chest pain, swollen joints, or frequent dizziness. I should point out that it is quite common to develop soreness after exercising, especially if you are new to increased physical activity. It's called DOMS, or delayed onset muscle soreness. It typically occurs twelve to seventy-two hours after strenuous activity. Try lifting too-heavy dumbbells or going too low on a bunch of squats and you will feel it. It usually is not related to underlying disease but rather represents your muscles remodeling—another reason to take it slow at first.

A couple of questions I want you to ask yourself when it comes to your personal heart disease prevention program: How important do you think it is for you to be physically active? And why do you think that?

That tells me almost everything. If you don't truly think exercise is important, you aren't going to make it a priority.

You need to create a relationship with exercise so that it's not a chore you need to check off but an activity that is part of your lifestyle. Make it a critical element of your personal heart disease prevention program. I always tell patients to focus on where they want to be a year from now and five years from now, not next month. By that I mean, it doesn't help much if you start off strong, exercising four days a week, and then burn out after two months. Rather, if exercise becomes a natural part of the way you live your life, it's a major win!

I wish doctors talked more about exercise when it comes to helping you reduce your heart disease risk. And I'm not talking about the perfunctory "you should go to the gym" or "you need to start exercising." Instead, we need to be writing exercise prescriptions.

**EXERCISE RX**

MON — Walk for 30 min & pilates

TUES – Weights at gym

WED – Walk for 30 min

THU – Walk for 30 min

FRI – Weights at gym

SAT – Walk for 30 min

SUN – REST DAY!

There's been a fair amount of discussion in recent years suggesting that whether or not one engages in exercise should be considered a vital sign—just like we measure heart rate, blood pressure, and weight. Exercise is about promoting your longevity—that's how important it is.

That's why I included as part of this book a four-week exercise plan to help you get started as well as keep you on track. (See appendix A.) It can be confusing and a little bit intimidating, especially when you are beginning an exercise program. I give you various exercises to choose from and show that you have to progress over time. It's a framework to help you along the way.

I often recommend to patients that they consider a personal trainer—either in-person or virtual—for a few sessions. This can help you choose the right exercises for your personal circumstance as well as keep you accountable. I know I always show up when I'm paying for something. Given the cost, this isn't practical for everyone. There are some free apps as well as numerous online sites that provide useful guidance. What I don't want you to do is buy some equipment or go to the gym and then try to figure out what to do. That's never a winning strategy. You don't have to use the plan at the end of the book, but you do need to have a plan.

---

## Summary

Engaging in an exercise program will help reduce your risk for heart disease. Aim for between seventy-five and two hundred minutes of exercise each week. Choose any type of physical activity that you like. Remember, exercise doesn't have to involve a trip to the gym. Make sure to do both aerobic activities as well as one or two sessions of strength training with weights, exercise machines, or even your own body weight. And don't forget to regularly up the intensity of your workouts. It's okay to include low- to moderate-intensity workouts in your routine. But try for at least two of your weekly workouts to be performed at a high or "vigorous" intensity, if you can tolerate it. And whatever you do, make sure it's something that you enjoy enough that you can sustain it for the long haul.

## ANSWERS

1. **True**. Even fifteen minutes of *daily* exercise adds up to benefits in reducing your risk for a heart attack. The key is to be consistent.

2. **True**. Exercise can help reduce cholesterol levels.

3. **False**. Although aerobic and strength training each reduce heart disease risk, doing both has the most benefit. It's important to incorporate both in your weekly exercise routine.

4. **True**. The reality is you do have to put forth some exertion to get the most benefit. This doesn't mean every exercise needs to be full exertion; even light exercise provides benefit, but some exertion helps.

5. **False**. Both exercise and diet are important in reducing risk, and we can't say that exercise is more important.

## CHAPTER EIGHT

# Supplements— Do They Work?

**TRUE OR FALSE?**

1. If supplements are in the store or sold online, they're basically safe.
2. Vitamin D plays an important role in heart health.
3. Fish oil supplements give the same benefit as eating fish.
4. Focusing on gut health helps your heart.
5. Garlic can help reduce cholesterol.

*(Answers at end of chapter)*

"WHAT DO YOU THINK ABOUT coenzyme Q10?"

"My neighbor takes vitamin D. She says I should be taking it too. Is that okay?"

"I really don't like fish. Aren't fish oil pills just as good?"

"There's no real harm to vitamins, so why not try them?"

These are some of the most common questions patients ask me about supplements. And I should point out, many patients probably don't tell me they are taking them because they don't think it's important to mention it. If you only remember one thing from this chapter (and I hope it's more than one!), it must be that you definitely need to tell your doctor and pharmacist if you are taking supplements. They can interact with prescription medications, changing their amount in your bloodstream—and that can sometimes cause problems.

Supplements and vitamins are a multibillion dollar business. It's really not surprising. To be fair, trying to eat healthy can be challenging. To make it easier, people often turn to a pill, capsule, bar, or powder with the hope that it can give the same benefit—or almost the same—as a healthy meal. Others just want to supplement to get an "extra edge." Seems reasonable, doesn't it? Well, it's a bit more complicated.

In general, I try to keep an open mind, but honestly, I am not a big proponent of most supplements for a variety of reasons. I think it can lull people into a false sense of security that if they pop a pill or scoop a powder, they can just eat whatever they want. In addition, the body does not metabolize supplements the same way it does whole foods. Despite you trying to convince yourself that swallowing a fish oil pill is the same as eating fish, the benefits just are not the same.

Full disclosure—I'm also likely influenced by my time working at the US Food and Drug Administration. Supplements are not regulated the same way drugs are— meaning that supplements do not need to undergo rigorous clinical trials to demonstrate safety and effectiveness before they can be sold in the US. Rather, supplements are considered a food, and therefore, they can be sold without having to conduct trials. They can only be removed if they are proven to cause harm. The FDA has established standards to ensure quality, strength, and purity. The supplement industry has had some "bad apples" that made health claims not supported by any evidence as well as others that have had problems with the purity of their manufacturing process. To be fair, this is a minority of the total industry, but we do need to recognize that it's not the same approval process as for prescription or over-the-counter medicines.

## What Does "Natural" Mean?

Don't be fooled into thinking *natural* means "safe." For instance, there are plenty of natural herbs that can negatively affect your liver or kidney at too high a dose. It also doesn't mean it has a health benefit. FDA considers *natural* to mean that nothing artificial or synthetic has been put into a food that wouldn't be expected to be there. It doesn't address food production, processing, or manufacturing methods.

## What's the Latest Data?

Numerous medical groups have studied the value of some vitamins and supplements to promote health over the last couple of decades. The most recent analysis was in June 2022. The United States Preventive Services Task Force updated its recommendation on the use of vitamins and supplements based on an evidence report that included more than eighty studies. The task force, an independent panel of national experts, found there was not enough evidence that supplements help prevent heart disease, stroke, or cancer. There was an exception of a small benefit with multivitamin use for cancer prevention.

The task force did not look at all supplements. Rather its report suggested that if you are a healthy, nonpregnant adult, there is "insufficient evidence" of any benefits to extending one's life by taking vitamin E, vitamin D, calcium, vitamin A, beta-carotene, vitamin $B_3$, vitamin $B_6$, vitamin C, or selenium. They also concluded with moderate certainty that there is no net benefit of supplementation with vitamin E for the prevention of cardiovascular disease or cancer.

In many ways, I find it rather surprising that the current evidence is insufficient. We have been studying vitamins and supplements for years. If something really worked as well as some people suggest, it would not be a secret. We would all know about it! Given the decades of research and the number of people using supplements, I'd expect that if there were benefit, we would know by now. Wouldn't you?

I do want to point out that "insufficient" doesn't mean conclusively that there is no benefit. Maybe it depends on whether you are a "glass half empty" or "glass half full" person. Your attitude might be, "Well, it might. So I should try it." That might be okay for a gadget in the house, but in health-care, we try to be fairly certain something works before we put it into our bodies. Again, we've had many years to study, and if there were a "magic pill," as some supplement companies try to suggest, we'd have found it by now.

There's also this common belief that since you can buy vitamins and supplements without prescriptions, they're harmless. Well, that's not always true.

In fact, the task force concluded with moderate certainty

that the harms of beta-carotene supplementation outweigh the benefits for the prevention of cardiovascular disease or cancer. Simply put, this means they could possibly increase risk of cardiovascular mortality and lung cancer. There was also limited evidence suggesting potential risks from some supplements, such as vitamin A being associated with higher risk of hip fracture, vitamin E being linked to hemorrhagic stroke, as well as increased cancer incidence from folic acid, and increased incidence of kidney stones from vitamin C and calcium.

As I mentioned earlier, the task force did not look at all supplements and vitamins. I also don't want you to think I am against every vitamin and supplement in every circumstance because that is not the case, especially for those people with documented nutritional deficiencies. While there is no replacement for high-quality whole foods, including the many that have been discussed throughout the book and that are highlighted in the meal plans in appendix B, there are some that I do wish to discuss given the number of questions I get on them.

**Probiotics.** We usually think of bacteria as something that can cause diseases or other problems. But good bacteria can help promote health. Probiotics are a type of "good" bacteria found in some foods and supplements. The reason why this might impact your health in a positive way is that they might lower the number of "bad" bacteria in your gut that can cause illness or inflammation. They basically crowd out the bad bacteria.

Sometimes patients take probiotics when they also take antibiotics to help with some of the diarrhea that can occur. When it comes to your heart, some data suggests probiotics can help lower LDL cholesterol, increase HDL cholesterol, and lower blood pressure—all of which help decrease your overall risk of heart disease.

Probiotics can be found in foods such as yogurt, kefir, kimchi, pickles, and sauerkraut. Many people I know consume them as supplements, which come in many different forms, including capsules, liquids, and pills. These are fragile bacteria in supplement form and usually need to be refrigerated.

Keep in mind that because you will be changing your gut bacteria, they can cause mild stomach problems, especially the first few days you start taking them. You might have stomach upset, gas, diarrhea, or bloating. In a small number of people, probiotics can trigger an allergic reaction. If you have an immune system problem or another serious health condition, you may have a greater chance of issues and you definitely should discuss with your doctor before you start consuming them as supplements.

**Garlic.** Coming from an Italian family, garlic was often around at dinner time. To this day, it is one of the most popular ingredients in cooking in many households. In case you are wondering, the unmistakable taste and aroma is due to a compound called allicin, which is an antioxidant that may benefit the heart.

For many years, we used to think garlic could help reduce total cholesterol and LDL, but most recent studies have not confirmed that. Some studies have shown that it helps to reduce blood pressure and blood sugar, but we need more studies to know that for sure.

I find that when people want to take a garlic supplement, they often are not aware of the high dose they are taking. I mention this because I don't think we've seen value in taking high doses. In addition, such usage can interact with some blood thinners, including aspirin, and cause heartburn.

Here's my advice on garlic: if you like garlic in your food, keep using it. But don't spend the money on pills or powders. Bonus tip: the best benefit comes when garlic is crushed or chopped!

**Fiber.** I talked about the benefits of a high-fiber diet earlier in the book. Fiber helps lower cholesterol as well as keeps your blood sugar stabilized. It helps you feel full so you don't overeat, reducing the chance for obesity. Insoluble fiber adds bulk to stools, which you probably know helps keep you "regular."

A number of studies have found that a high intake of total fiber, from foods and supplements, lowers the risk of heart disease. High-fiber diets have also been associated with a reduced risk of type 2 diabetes.

Current recommendations are that women should try to eat at least 21 to 25 grams of fiber a day, while men should aim for 30 to 38 grams a day. However, most of us only consume about half of the recommended amount.

That's where fiber supplementation may play a role. There are various forms, including capsules and powders. There are even wafer-type cookies and gummies. Personally, I eat a fiber wafer several days a week, especially if I'm having trouble getting the recommended amount in food.

Of course, I don't want you to avoid eating fiber-rich foods in lieu of a powder, but if you do have trouble incorporating enough fiber into your diet, supplementation may be helpful.

**Omega-3 fatty acids.** Omega-3 fatty acids are nutrients (polyunsaturated fats, to be exact!) that you get through food or supplements that may be important for preventing and managing heart disease. The main benefit seems to be the potential role in lowering triglycerides and blood pressure—both of which decrease heart risk. They also may reduce inflammation that can damage the lining of our blood vessels. That can translate into lower blood pressure. Two crucial omega-3s—EPA and DHA—are primarily found in certain fish, which is why omega-3s are sometimes referred to as "fish oils." They are particularly crucial because our bodies don't make them naturally.

Salmon, sardines, herring, mackerel, and canned tuna are among the most common sources of fish oil.

I often get asked by people who don't like eating fish if they can just pop a fish pill instead and get the same benefit. Sometimes patients will suggest to me that fish oil capsules are better than eating fish since there's no mercury or other toxins. I tend to agree with the American Heart Association, and they say that to get the maximum omega-3 fatty acid health benefit, you need to eat fish since it has cardiovascular benefit but also healthy vitamins and minerals, as well as protein that you just can't get from fish oil supplements.

You should also be aware some recent data suggests high doses of fish oil supplements (typically more than 1 gram) may increase the risk of atrial fibrillation, an abnormal heart rhythm.

I should point out there are also omega-3 prescriptions available for adults with triglycerides 500 mg/dL or above. Unlike fish oil supplements, these medications are approved and monitored for quality and safety by the FDA for specific use.

**Turmeric**. Most likely sitting in your spice drawer is turmeric, a common spice used in cooking as well as making drinks. Turmeric has been around and used for medicinal purposes for hundreds of years because of its anti-inflammatory properties. As we discussed in earlier chapters, inflammation is a big topic of interest since chronic inflammation can cause many undesirable health outcomes, such as heart disease. It is believed that the property in turmeric called curcumin may be responsible for helping to lower heart disease risk. Curcumin is a potent antioxidant that can neutralize free radicals due to its chemical structure. That helps protect your blood vessels from getting damaged and allowing plaques to rupture.

In addition to turmeric's anti-inflammatory properties, it appears this supplement can help lower LDL (bad) cholesterol and triglycerides. Results have been encouraging, but we still need more data to know.

As I keep mentioning, supplements can interact with prescription medicines, so check with your doctor before taking turmeric supplements if you're taking blood thinners, such as warfarin. Like garlic, I suggest to patients if you like using it as part of your food, that's great. We need a bit more data before we start ingesting turmeric pills.

**CoQ10.** Coenzyme Q10 (CoQ10) is a nutrient that occurs naturally in the body. CoQ10 is also in many foods we eat. Like some other supplements, CoQ10 acts as an antioxidant, which protects cells from damage.

Although CoQ10 plays a key role in the body, most healthy people have enough CoQ10 naturally. There is some evidence that adding more—in the form of CoQ10 supplements—may be beneficial. As we get older and develop health problems, CoQ10 levels seem to drop. But in these cases, it's uncertain that adding CoQ10 will have an effect.

There's some emerging evidence that CoQ10 supplements can lower blood pressure slightly. CoQ10 is also used to treat heart failure and other heart conditions, possibly helping to improve some symptoms and lessen future cardiac risks when combined with regular medications, but the evidence is conflicting.

You've likely also heard of CoQ10 if you are on certain medications to treat cholesterol. Some doctors even recommend it as a treatment for the side effects of statins. Why? Statins can sometimes lower the amount of CoQ10 the body makes on its own. Some doctors suggest adding a CoQ10 supplement to make up for the loss, hoping it will relieve problems like muscle pain and weakness. But overall scientific evidence does not support the use of CoQ10 for muscle pain caused by statins.

**Vitamin D**. I know many people take vitamin D for different reasons. It helps with our bones as well as our overall immune function. But when it comes to your heart, research has been mixed on any health benefits. We've seen when there is a documented vitamin D deficiency, there seems to be an association with high blood pressure and heart disease. But when these patients were given vitamin D, it's not clear supplementation improved their health.

Like many other vitamins and supplements, the data is mixed—some show heart benefit; some show none. Yet we do know vitamin D remains an important nutrient for overall good health. The National Academies of Sciences, Engineering, and Medicine recommends 600 international units (IU) of vitamin D a day for adults aged nineteen to seventy. For adults age seventy-one and older, the recommendation increases to 800 IU a day.

I always recommend to patients to first get their level

checked. If it's normal, supplementation usually isn't necessary. Remember, fifteen to thirty minutes of sunlight most days of the week also can help maintain vitamin D levels.

**Calcium**. When discussing vitamin D with patients, I always try to also bring up calcium. Some people take calcium supplements as part of a strategy to prevent osteoporosis. Because there is some data that suggests calcium supplementation might be associated with increased risk of heart disease, it's a good idea to also take vitamin D in combination with the calcium. This may decrease any adverse events. Interestingly, research does not suggest that calcium from whole foods is associated with any increased risk—just the supplements. This is an area of continuing research.

**Magnesium**. Magnesium and its relationship to the heart have been studied for decades. Magnesium deficiency has been linked to high blood pressure, stroke, diabetes, and even osteoporosis. As a resident at Duke University, I was part of some studies of its use in the cardiac care unit. Some of the strongest data in recent years relates to its impact on our heart rhythm—how well it beats. Magnesium also might help keep blood pressure in the normal range, and this may be why it is purported to lower risk of heart attacks.

Food can be a great source of magnesium if you know what to eat. I discussed this earlier. An easy way to remember foods that are good magnesium sources is to think of fiber. Foods that are high in fiber are generally also high in magnesium. Dietary sources of magnesium include legumes, whole grains, wheat germ, oat bran, vegetables (especially broccoli and squash), seeds, and nuts (especially almonds).

As with other important minerals, some people do

not get enough magnesium through food alone and could consider supplementation. If you're healthy, your kidneys flush out the extra magnesium, so consuming too much is unusual. Some conditions, such as myasthenia gravis, can get worse if you take too much magnesium. Again, it's important to talk to your doctor before you start supplementation.

I also want to remind you that more is not usually better. I find when people start supplements, they often increase doses—thinking that if a little helps, taking more might even work better. That's usually not the case and can even put one at risk. For example, vitamin D supplementation at 400 IU to 1,000 IU daily showed improvement, but at 4,000 IU daily, there was a decrease in bone mineral density and lower strength.

---

## Summary

There are no magic pills or powders to prevent heart disease. From a nutrition standpoint, a healthy, well-balanced diet is the best way to reduce your risk of heart disease. If you do have nutritional deficiencies, it can be helpful to talk to your doctor or a nutritionist as to what supplementation might be appropriate for you since some supplements can be valuable to your health. Don't take supplements in place of or in combination with prescription medications unless you first talk to your health-care provider.

## ANSWERS

1. **False**. Supplements are regulated as a food and do not have to undergo any trials for safety and efficacy.

2. **True**. Vitamin D plays an important role in our bodies, including supporting bone health, immune function, and heart health.

3. **False**. Swallowing a fish oil pill can have some benefits, but it does not have the same benefits as eating a piece of fish.

4. **True**. Gut health plays a role in heart health. Taking care of your gastrointestinal tract has benefits for your body overall, including your heart.

5. **False**. Right now, we just don't know for sure whether garlic truly lowers cholesterol.

## CHAPTER NINE

# The Role of Medication

---

### TRUE OR FALSE?

1. If you adopt a healthy lifestyle, you don't need medications to prevent heart disease.
2. Everyone should be on a baby aspirin after age fifty.
3. When it comes to heart disease, being on a statin to lower cholesterol has more benefits than risks.
4. Managing diabetes and high blood pressure with meds can reduce your risk of heart disease.
5. The recommended use of medications doesn't differ whether you are trying to prevent the first heart attack or a second one.

*(Answers at end of chapter)*

---

TERRI IS SIXTY YEARS OLD. She has high blood pressure but otherwise is in pretty good health. Her recent colonoscopy screening was normal. She tries to be active at least three days of the week, and she is a big proponent of quality sleep. She is very engaged in her care and often sends me questions via secure messaging. Recently, she sent me this query: "Hey, Dr. Whyte. Should I be on an aspirin? I remember my mother was on one. Just wanted to check."

I love the fact that Terri asks lots of questions. And I encourage you to do that too. And if your doctor doesn't like all your questions, find another doctor!

As for Terri's question, five years ago, I might have given her a different answer than I would give today. That's because based on much more research and looking at her underlying health, and the fact that she has not had a heart attack, the answer for her is that she doesn't need to be on aspirin.

For years, we thought everyone needed to be on aspirin—at least a low dose (often referred to as "baby aspirin," since the dose is 81 mg instead of the more typical 325 mg)—whether or not they had heart disease. My mother was on aspirin for years. But like some others, she developed bleeding in her colon and had to stop taking it. The reason to put her on aspirin in the first place has changed based on new research.

Aspirin serves many purposes, but when it comes to your heart, it's mostly about the impact on platelets. Aspirin helps to make platelets less sticky. When aspirin stops platelets from being sticky, it can reduce the risk of a clot that can cause a heart attack, but it can also increase bleeding elsewhere in the body, which can be very serious.

It's a balance. When it comes to aspirin use to prevent heart attacks, you need to ask a couple questions. The first question is: What's your underlying risk? This mostly depends on age and whether or not you've already had a heart attack. The second question is: What's my risk of too much bleeding? Remember, this book is all about primary *prevention*—meaning you have not already had a heart attack. The information here about aspirin and other medications does not apply if you've already had a heart attack.

---

## Current Aspirin Recommendations

Who does the current recommendations apply to?

- If you are between forty and fifty-nine and have a 10 percent or higher risk of developing heart disease in ten years (remember I mentioned those risk calculators in chapter 3?), daily low-dose aspirin use provides a small net benefit. If your risk is lower, you likely do not need a daily aspirin.
- Your doctor might also suggest aspirin if you're younger than sixty and you have diabetes and at least one other heart disease risk factor, such as smoking or high blood pressure.
- If you're sixty years of age or older, aspirin use for primary prevention has no net benefit.

I do need to point out that if you are currently taking aspirin for primary prevention and you don't fit these new recommendations, do *not* stop taking it. Rather, talk to your doctor about it.

Throughout the book, I've been discussing ways to reduce your personal risk of heart disease. Even though I have spent the last several chapters on lifestyle changes, some of you will also need medication to reduce the risk further, especially for those risk factors that play a big role in heart disease.

## Drugs for Diabetes

I mentioned early on that having diabetes has a multiplier effect on your risk of heart disease. That means it dramatically increases your risk of heart disease (and some other conditions) compared to if you didn't have diabetes. As a result, managing your blood sugar levels and getting them as close to the normal range as possible will help reduce your risk of a heart attack. For a variety of reasons, everyone won't be able to do this adequately with diet and lifestyle, so medications can play an important role.

What's particularly interesting is that in the last couple of years, we've seen several new medications for the treatment of type 2 diabetes that also can reduce risk of heart disease. They work through different mechanisms but have the same effect on risk. The first is a class of drugs called sodium-glucose cotransporter-2 (SGLT2) inhibitors that lower blood sugar by helping the body excrete it in urine. They also prevent excess fluid from building up in the body, which reduces the risk of developing heart failure.

The second is an injectable drug known as glucagon-like peptide-1 receptor agonists (GLP-1). It helps your pancreas release the proper amount of insulin to keep blood sugar levels in check. But it also makes you feel full longer, can lead to weight loss, and reduces your risk of having a heart attack or stroke.

Some of you with diabetes reading this book may not be on these medications. Be sure to talk to your doctor if these newer medications are right for you. They can be more expensive, and sometimes insurance companies don't pay for them or force you to try older medications first. Don't take no for an answer if your doctor thinks these are right for your diabetes management because they will also reduce your heart disease risk. This is relatively new information and not everyone may be aware of it, including your doctor.

***

## Cholesterol-Lowering Medications

By now, most people know that high cholesterol can increase your risk of heart disease. Whether or not you can manage by diet alone or should be on medication for primary prevention relates to risk. Notice the theme in this chapter: evaluating the risks versus benefits of medications.

You may not realize that statins don't just reduce bad cholesterol and raise good cholesterol. Some also help prevent blood clots as well as inflammation, which also reduces the risk of a heart attack.

The current primary prevention recommendation for starting medication to lower cholesterol to prevent a heart attack is as follows:

- If you are between ages forty to seventy-five and have a ten-year risk of heart disease that is 7.5 percent or higher (we discussed how to calculate risk in chapter 3).
- If you are between forty and seventy-five years of age and you have type 2 diabetes.
- If you have LDL cholesterol levels of 190 mg/dL (4.92 mmol/L) or higher. This is a rather high number and sometimes indicates a condition called familial hypercholesterolemia, which significantly increases your heart disease risk.

Statins also lower the stiffness of your arteries and slow the progression of such stiffness. Remember, keeping your blood vessels open and flexible is a good thing. Like all drugs, statins can cause side effects. These can include upset stomach, brown urine, muscle pain, and liver damage. Your doctor will order some lab tests to make sure none of these become serious. In recent years, we have noticed that some patients with diabetes can see their blood sugars rise slightly, so that also needs to be monitored. We also need to assess if statin usage increases the future risk of developing diabetes.

If you haven't already asked your doctor, be sure to find out whether they recommend that you take a statin to help reduce your risk for heart attack and stroke. Make sure they tell you why or why not. Don't assume that if you aren't on one now that you don't need to be on one. You may or may not, but you want to know the reasons.

## Blood Pressure Medications

If you want to control your heart disease risk, you need to control your blood pressure. Although some people can control their high blood pressure through diet and lifestyle changes, others will need medications. We used to think that blood pressure medications only helped people with already-established heart disease. But recent studies have shown that treating blood pressure with medication plays a role in primary prevention of heart disease too. There's even some recent data that taking blood pressure medications at night might have more benefits to your heart. Of course, talk to your doctor before you make any changes in your medications. There are lots of choices for blood pressure medication—and you want to make sure you are taking one that can play a role in reducing risk for heart disease, either directly or indirectly.

---

## Questions to Ask

With any medication to help reduce your risk of heart disease—whether it's directly or indirectly—you want to ask questions. At a minimum, you should ask the following:

- Why am I taking it?
- Will I need to take it for the rest of my life?
- What are the potential side effects?
- How do I know if the medication is working?
- Are there any special instructions for taking this medication (e.g., with meals, on an empty stomach, in the morning, in the evening)?
- Are there any activities I should avoid while taking it?
- Is there any new data I should be aware of?

This book is all about what you can do to reduce your risk of heart disease. Sometimes, medications play a role. I don't want you to think that if you need to take medication, that means lifestyle changes don't work. Based on your personal risk and other health conditions, you might need more help than lifestyle changes alone can provide. Lifestyle changes may mean a lower dose of medication or even fewer medications than you might have needed if you were not taking control of your risk. Of course, starting medications doesn't mean you can stop your healthy eating, physical activity, stress reduction, and quality sleep. They all play a role in your heart health.

---

## Summary

Medications can play an important role in reducing your risk of heart disease. Their role differs depending on whether the goal is to prevent a first heart attack or a second heart attack. It's especially critical to treat high blood pressure and high cholesterol—and sometimes these need medication along with lifestyle changes. Be sure to ask your doctor specific questions about your heart before you start or stop any medicine.

---

### ANSWERS

1. **False**. Although lifestyle changes play a key role in reducing your risk of heart disease, some people will still need to take medicines to further reduce risk.

2. **False**. Whether or not you are on an aspirin after the age of fifty depends on your overall health, with a careful discussion with your doctor on the risks and benefits of aspirin. Years ago, we thought everyone should be on aspirin after age fifty, but we no longer believe that.

3. **True**. For many people, using a statin to lower cholesterol gives more benefits than risks in reducing heart disease.

4. **True**. Since high blood pressure and diabetes are major risk factors for diabetes, taking medications to treat them can help reduce your risk of having a heart attack.

5. **False**. There is a significant difference in how we assess medication risk and benefit for people who do not already have heart disease (primary prevention) versus those who already have heart disease (secondary prevention).

# CONCLUSION

## Putting It All Together

CONGRATULATIONS! YOU DID IT! NINE chapters and you are still reading about what you can do to reduce your heart disease risk. We've covered a lot of material:

- Take a good family history.
- Calculate your risk score.
- Get the right laboratory and diagnostic tests.
- Stay up-to-date on screening exams.
- Eat more fruits and vegetables.
- Drink mostly water.
- Be active four days a week.
- Screen for depression.
- Reduce your stress.

When you list out everything we've talked about over the last nine chapters, it can seem a bit daunting. "Dr. Whyte, I have to do all that?" For many of you, it will be a lot to address. But I assure you the benefits of making these lifestyle changes are well worth the time and effort. Remember, most diseases—including heart disease—are caused by lifestyle. Adopt a healthy lifestyle and you reduce your risk.

You've already taken a key step in reducing your risk by getting informed. There's a lot of misinformation out there in terms of what you need to do in order to reduce your heart risk, especially as it relates to nutrition, exercise, and mental health. But now you are well informed and ready to take action. Knowledge is power, and you should feel powerful! You've jumped over a main hurdle, which is not knowing what to do. Now that you have the information, how do you make healthy living a priority? How do you enact meaningful change?

One of my goals in writing this book is to also show that living a healthy lifestyle is *not* boring. Sometimes people think making healthy choices is all about denying yourself tasty treats and fun. "I can't say up late." "I can't drink alcohol." "You're taking away ice cream." I'm not suggesting you can't do those things. You just can't do them every day or most days of the week. Adopting new behaviors can be incredibly enjoyable. Try new foods with new flavors; experiment with different activities that get you going in the morning; use mindfulness to improve your mood and wake up well rested.

There's a new phrase that I want you to be aware of: "Health happens outside the doctor's office." By this I mean what you do when you are at home determines your overall health, much more so than what your blood pressure or heart rate is when you get them checked at the doctor's office. Sure, it matters what happens during your appointment. But what I really care about is what you are doing every day—what you are eating, whether you are addressing stress and depression, how active you are. These are the critical components to reducing your risk of heart disease.

You also need to recognize that you have a big role to play in your own care. Of course, the doctor plays an important role. But you play the bigger role. It's your life, and you want to do what you can to maximize how long and how well you live. The information in each of the chapters gives its own benefit, but when combined together, it all packs a powerful punch in reducing risk.

I recognize that making changes can be difficult—some more so than others. And there will be starts and stops. That's the normal process in change. The key is to get started!

I do want to offer a few tips I've learned over the years.

- **Don't tackle too many things at once.** People often get excited about what they can do to lower their risk, and they try to do too much at once. That's a recipe for disaster. Instead, start with one or maybe two things. For example, start eating fish twice a week or stop eating after 7:00 p.m. Or commit to exercising twenty minutes three times a week. Make change evolutionary, not revolutionary! It's hard for your mind and body to process too many changes all at once. Choose one or two things at a time and then add more as you progress through your health journey.

- **Make short- and long-term goals.** And by short, that often means a daily action plan at the beginning. What's your goal today? Drink five glasses of water?

Do meditation for ten minutes? Eat a piece of fruit? Goals need to be explicit, and you need an action plan to get to them. Don't just say "I'm going to eat healthy." Rather, make a plan of how you are going to do it. That means, for example, making sure you have a water bottle when you're out and about. It means stocking your pantry with healthy foods and getting rid of the processed ones. It means blocking the time on your schedule to do meditation and make it a priority.

- **Track progress.** This will allow you to stay focused and self-monitor. A good example is having a weight loss goal of a pound a week. You track progress by weighing yourself. But as I've said before, I don't think you need to weigh yourself every day. Instead, I would do it twice a week, and as you progress in your goals, once a week and then every two weeks. Feedback is important as you make changes, but it needs to be the right type and right frequency. I don't want you to get frustrated or disappointed if you don't see progress every day. You're in it for the long haul. Tracking progress will help. I also like it because you want to make sure you don't get off track for too many days in a row, so that's why it's important to track several times a week but not every day.

- **Enlist others.** Telling other people about your goals as well as connecting with others who are working on similar goals can increase accountability and make you more likely to succeed. Some people find it fun to work with friends on common goals, and others believe it's important to share goals with family members to help encourage new behaviors. It doesn't need to be many people. Even just one person who can help encourage you, as well as be a good "sounding board," can be every effective in helping you sustain lifestyle changes. This can be especially helpful if you live with others. It can be hard to eat healthy when one partner or spouse focuses on junk food; making healthy living a family activity can help not just you but your loved ones as well!

- **Be patient.** Change requires time. It took a while to develop unhealthy habits—and it will take a while to undevelop them. Change doesn't happen overnight, despite your best intentions. I always tell people I'm less interested in how you are doing three months from now or six months from now versus how you are doing a year from now, three years from now, ten years from now. I want to see the long-term success, not the typical weight loss for summer!

One of the biggest mistakes I see is that people start all motivated to make change and then, as my patient Leslie likes to say, "Life gets in the way." My response to comments like this has always been that you don't have to be perfect every day. Some days, you wake up feeling lousy and you eat too much fast food. Guess what? That's okay. It's the daily choices over time that matter. Your goal is to have many more healthy days of the month and only one or two not-so-healthy days.

I also want to point out that when it comes to heart health, there is a lot of research being conducted. Therefore, it's important to stay up-to-date on the latest information—whether it's nutrition, exercise, lab tests, or medications.

It's also critical to create partnerships with your primary care physician, nurse practitioner, and pharmacist. You need to ask the following questions every year:

1. What should I be doing to reduce my risk for heart disease?
2. Are there any lab tests I need today?
3. Are there any imaging studies or other diagnostic tests I need?
4. Should I be on any medications to reduce my risk, or should I change medication?
5. Do you have any concerns about how I'm doing?
6. Do you need to refer me to anyone?

Let's admit it. Doctors are too rushed during most visits. They don't always address all issues in as much detail as they should. All too often, prevention strategies get missed. That's why you also can play a role in bringing them up. Your risk will change as you age and develop other health conditions. Don't assume the advice you were given five years ago still applies today. Ask the questions—and if your doctor doesn't answer them or gets annoyed at your asking them, then find a new doctor.

Your heart is an amazing organ. I don't want you to ignore it until it starts to develop problems. You need to take care of it now to prevent damage, or at least delay it. Remember—you have the power to reduce your risk of heart disease. Use it.

# ACKNOWLEDGMENTS

THIS BOOK IS THE THIRD in a series that promotes one's ability to take control of one's own health. I'm enormously grateful to have had the opportunity to communicate this information on heart disease in new and creative ways.

None of this would have been possible without my literary agent, Mel Berger, who convinced me that I needed to write these books because of the potential to impact lives in meaningful ways. That has been my goal—empower consumers with credible, practical information so they can live a healthier and longer life. Thanks, Mel, for making this happen.

I appreciate the input from folks who graciously agreed to read various drafts. Both my sisters, Charlene and Jackie, helped me write in ways that wasn't all scientific jargon. My colleagues at WebMD—James Beckerman, MD; Brunilda Nazario, MD; Neha Pathak, MD; Beth Passehl; and Bethany Afshar—made sure my recommendations were backed by published research. My good friend Anahad O'Connor helped me organize my thoughts through his unique ability to debate data in an educational and fun process!

Dr. Christopher Mohr has helped me learn some of the key principles of nutrition over the past two decades, and I try to put them into practice every day. I've shared many in this book. I also want to express appreciation to Greg Herrell, an extraordinary personal trainer and certified strength conditioning specialist who knows how to use the mechanics of exercise to improve the way the heart functions. We both like to remind people that fitness is about longevity more than it is about appearance.

I'm profoundly grateful to Dr. Phil McGraw, Ph.D. Dr. Phil and I have had many conversations about the connection between mental health and heart health. These discussions led to a focus on mental health and stress as key risk factors that need to be addressed.

For a book like this to be successful, it can't just be words. There needs to be pictures as well. My gratitude to Emily Berry as well as Vella Torres who jumped into action to create graphics in record time. Their work helped communicate some of my most important points in ways that grab one's attention.

It's not possible to talk or write about the heart and not think about love. Writing a book is truly a family affair given the amount of time it takes. Thank you to the three loves of my life—Alisa, Luke, and Jack—for all their support and encouragement.

Finally, I want to express my gratitude to Emilio Pardo, who always encouraged me to become active in the media and communications world. Emilio was a rarity in Washington, DC, with his constant optimism, relentless focus on purpose, and a unique ability to help people reimagine their lives. Cancer took him too soon, but his impact on many people, including me, remains.

# Sample Exercise Plan

EXERCISE IS ESSENTIAL TO A heart disease prevention program. Following is a general four-week plan to help you get started in terms of what you can do and for how often. The exercises here are based on a variety of factors. This plan can serve as a foundation for you.

The structure of the four-week plan is as follows: four days weekly total, with two days of cardiovascular/flexibility training and two days of resistance/core training. Ideally, you will spend forty-five to sixty minutes per session, but starting with less and working up to this amount is a good strategy as well. On the days you are not training, feel free to get in some form of active recovery, such as walking; just make sure whatever you choose is not too strenuous so the body has time to rest and repair.

---

## Week 1, Day 1: Resistance Training/Core

### Step-Ups

These can be done with or without added weight, depending on the height of the step and your ability/strength. Make sure whatever you use as your step is safe and stable to step on.

Sets/Reps: 3 sets of 10 reps.

1. Stand tall with your feet shoulder-width apart and facing the structure you will be stepping onto.
2. Lift your right leg and place your foot on the step structure you've chosen, keeping your ankle, knee, and hip in a straight alignment.
3. As your foot is being placed on the step, drive your weight into the middle of your foot to raise yourself forward and onto your step. As you step, make sure you keep yourself upright and tall.
4. Place your left foot next to your right foot and stand all the way up.
5. Remove your right leg first, followed by your left leg, and return both to their starting positions.
6. Repeat 10 reps on one leg at a time, then switch sides and repeat 10 times on the opposite leg.

**Pro Tip:** To get other muscles involved, try a "lateral step-up," which allows your body to move in a different plane of motion.

### Horizontal Rows

For those of us who sit all day (often hunched over), or even those who don't, it's important we incorporate "pulling" our back muscles into our routine. Examples of items to use are a gallon jug of water or a light (e.g., five- to ten-pound) dumbbell.

Sets/Reps: 3 sets of 10 reps on each arm. Rest for 30–90 seconds.

1. Using a chair or table, find a surface that is stable and about as tall as the height of your navel or hips.
2. Place one hand flat on the surface.
3. Hinging at your hips and keeping a neutral spine (straight back), bend over until your flat back is about 45 degrees relative to your hips.
4. With your opposite hand, grab the "weight" of your choosing; as an example, use a gallon jug of water.
5. Keeping your back at the 45-degree and neutral position, "row" the jug of water to your torso, making sure your elbow gets to a position of 90 degrees, ideally, and making sure to keep the elbow close to the body.
6. Pause for half a second and then extend your elbow and lower the jug back to the starting position, making sure to keep your torso from moving and not use any momentum to jerk the weight into position.

**Pro Tip:** Remember, you can always change the tempo of the exercise, slow it down or speed it up, increase time under tension, and make the exercise easier or more challenging.

### Hip Hinge

You do not want to neglect your lower body posterior chain muscles, so next up we have a hinge. A hinge can be done with your body weight, but making sure you are using proper form and sequencing here will be the key.

Sets/Reps: 3 sets of 10 reps.

1. Stand tall with your feet approximately shoulder-width apart and toes pointing forward (slightly everted, or out, is okay if it feels more comfortable).

2. Place your hands on your hips and pull (retract) your shoulders straight back as if you were trying to pinch something with your upper back.

3. Soften your knees very slightly and then make sure they do not travel any farther forward for the rest of the exercise.

4. Push your pelvis backwards as if you were a tea kettle tipping water into a cup. Another way to think about it is to imagine that as you're keeping your knees in that slightly bent position, you are pushing your butt back toward an imaginary wall.

5. Make sure as you begin lowering yourself you keep your back in that pinched position so that your back muscles stay "turned on."

6. As you get lower, you should start to feel a stretch in the back of your legs (hamstrings/glutes).

7. Stop yourself when you feel you lose that tension or recognize you're starting to now bend forward without keeping a straight/neutral spine. At that point, you've gone too far.

8. Stop yourself just before that position so that your posterior leg muscles stay engaged. Push your pelvis forward slowly, maintain your back position, and stand back up, squeezing your glutes, or butt muscles, at the top.

9. Repeat.

**Pro Tip:** Once you feel you've mastered the body weight hinge, try implementing a Romanian deadlift. Find a balanced object like a kettlebell or a case of bottled water and use this to add resistance to the exercise. Make sure you stop at your current end range of motion, or in other words, the point at which when you're lowering yourself you can no longer maintain a neutral spine position.

### Standing Curl to Overhead Press

Upper-body strength is important for a variety of reasons, but one that often comes into play is being able to lift luggage into overhead compartments. Use whatever weights you have at your disposal—dumbbells, soup cans, milk jugs—and make sure they are similar weight if you don't have a single, fixed object. Use caution if you have an existing or previous shoulder injury. Use pain as an indicator of caution.

Sets/Reps: 3 sets of 10 reps. Rest for 30–90 seconds.

1. Standing on a flat surface and making sure your feet are even with each other, curl your weight to your shoulders so that your elbows are at a 90-degree angle.
2. Keeping your elbows tucked in so that they run parallel to the sides of your body, press the objects overhead fully, extending your elbows.
3. At the top, a good check to make sure you're in a good position is to see if your biceps are in line with your ears.
4. Slowly lower the objects back down until your elbows reach about 90 degrees, and then press

back up again using control. Make sure to keep from using momentum to help, and don't lean back excessively.

5. Lower the weights back to the sides of your body, making sure to come all the way down so the weights rest next to your hips with your arms fully extended.

**Pro Tip:** Be sure to stay nice and tall without leaning backwards excessively. An excessive lean is often an indicator of too heavy of weight. At the top of the movement, your biceps should be right next to your ears.

### Plank

Core strength is crucial for protecting the spine, improves balance/stability, and allows the body to move optimally. A plank allows you to strengthen the core without unnecessary action of the spine (like in a sit-up), which many of us are not ready for if we are new to exercise. Find a pillow or something soft to rest your elbows on.

Sets/Reps: 3 sets of 30 seconds.
Rest for 30–90 seconds.

1. Get on the floor on all fours, positioning your elbows on the ground underneath your shoulders.
2. Extend your legs back so that you are balanced on your forearms and toes. Feet should be shoulder-width apart. Your body should be in a straight line from head to toe without sagging in the middle or arching your back.
3. Contract (create tension in) your core by pushing your forearms and feet hard into the ground.

4. Continue creating tension as you hold this position for 30 seconds.

**Pro Tip:** To make it more challenging on your core and upper body, try a plank to push-up. Continue switching back and forth from a plank to push-up for the same time period.

### Sumo Squat

A potentially safer alternative to a regular squat for those who don't have the mobility to get into the proper position, a sumo squat is similar to your "normal" squat, just with a wider stance. The sumo squat also can be done using a "low hold," which helps folks who have shoulder pain and lower back pain.

Sets/Reps: 3 sets of 12 reps. Rest for 30–90 seconds.

1. Spread your legs out about 6–12 inches wider than your shoulders on each side and point your toes about 45 degrees outward.
2. Keeping the weight of your body primarily on your heels and your back as upright as you can, lower your hips and allow your knees to bend into a wide squat.
3. Lower yourself so your quads are 90 degrees relative to your shins, or as close to this position as you can.
4. Squeeze your glutes as you start to stand back up.
5. At the top, be sure to stay tall and not overextend past your normal upright standing position.

**Pro Tip:** Try changing the tempo of the downward or upward motion to increase the difficulty, especially if you don't have enough weight to make the exercise challenging.

### Horizontal Floor Press

A floor press allows for upper-body horizontal pressing power without the need for a bench. Further, it increases focus on the upper body since the spine is in a fixed position and the elbows cannot travel past 90 degrees. Similar to the overhead press, find similarly weighted objects that can be safely held. Dumbbells would be ideal here, but any similarly weighted objects that can be utilized safely fit the criteria.

Sets/Reps: 3 sets of 12 reps. Rest for 30–90 seconds.

1. Grab a pair of dumbbells and lie down with your back and feet flat on the floor and your knees bent.
2. Take your dumbbells and position your arms at a 45-degree angle in relation to the side of your body with the dumbbells in your hands and your elbows on the floor.
3. Keeping your core tight and lower back in contact with the ground, press the dumbbells straight up until your arms are fully extended.
4. Lower the dumbbells with control (should take about two seconds to lower) until your elbows touch the ground.
5. Briefly pause for about one second before repeating the process.

**Pro Tip:** Try pressing one arm at a time for increased focus on pressing mechanics and to get the core more involved by stabilizing the weight.

## Week 1, Day 2: Cardiovascular Training/Flexibility

### *Aerobic Exercise*

30–60 minutes of aerobic-style exercise. Choose an activity you enjoy, such as walking, jogging, swimming, boxing, or cycling. On this day you will be focusing on aerobic exercise, which is a more steady-state form of cardio in which the intensity should be able to be sustained for 30–60 minutes continuously. Depending on your fitness level, it could be a walk or it may be a run. To help decide what's right for you, you should be able to have somewhat of a conversation at this intensity.

**Pro Tip:** Monitor your heart rate over time during and after exercise to see if you start to recover quicker as you get more efficient at aerobic cardio. Also monitor your resting heart rate; as you improve, your heart shouldn't have to beat as often to pump blood through your body. (This is a good thing, and it does take time to reach this level of fitness!)

### *Supine Active Hamstring Stretch*

Lots of people have tight hamstrings and hips, especially after activity. Having increased flexibility/mobility helps you to perform optimally and without pain when exercising.

Sets/Reps: 2 sets of 45 seconds on each leg. Rest after the second set as needed. Shoot for 30–90 seconds.

1. Lie on your back with both of your knees bent and feet on the floor.

2. Grab the back of your right thigh and pull your right knee toward your body.
3. Keeping your hands on the back of your right knee, extend your right leg until you feel a moderate stretch in your hamstring, and hold.
4. Pull your toes toward your shin to accentuate the stretch.
5. Switch legs.

**Pro Tip:** Use a towel or band if you find it hard to reach or hold your hands on the back of your knee.

### Superman Stretch

This move helps to mobilize the spine, open up the chest/sternum, and improve posture.

Sets/Reps: 2 sets of 12 reps.

1. Lie face down on your stomach and extend your arms and legs as far as you can.
2. Lift your arms, upper back, and legs off the floor as high as you can. Hold for 3 seconds, and then return to the floor.

**Pro Tip**: Consider holding a band to help add increased focus on improving your shoulder mobility as well.

_____

## Week 1, Day 3: Resistance Training/Core

### Walking Lunges

This is a great lower-body exercise that has elements of balance/stability since you are primarily using one leg at a time. Given that you will be using one leg at a time, you won't need as much external weight to create the desired training effect as you might for a more bilateral exercise (two legs at once) like a squat. If just using your body weight feels too difficult, try substituting with a bilateral movement until you build enough strength to use one leg at a time.

Sets/Reps: 3 sets of 8 reps/steps on each leg.
1. Stand tall, feet even with each other and shoulder-width apart.
2. Step forward a couple of feet with your right leg and plant your foot while simultaneously bending your right knee and lowering yourself down into a lunge position.
3. Without moving your right foot, stand back up and repeat the same motion on your left leg.
4. Try to keep moving forward without much pause during reps.

**Pro Tip:** Pause in between steps until you master the ability to go from one step directly to the next.

### Push-Up/Incline Push-Up

Depending on your strength and mobility levels, you can make these as difficult or as easy as needed. To make it more challenging, change the tempo during the up or down portion of the exercise. To make it more manageable, change the angle of the push-up: in general, the higher and more acute the angle, the easier it will be to perform. Use a wall, a table, a countertop, or some type of sturdy furniture.

Sets/Reps: 3 sets of 10 reps.

1. Get on the floor on all fours, positioning your hands underneath or slightly wider than your shoulders.

2. Extend your legs back so that you are balanced on your hands and toes. Feet should be shoulder-width apart. Your body should be in a straight line from head to toe without sagging in the middle or arching your back.

3. Contract (create tension), corkscrew your hands into the ground clockwise, push back into your toes, and brace your core. (Imagine what you would do with your body if you were outside in a hurricane—get tight!)

4. Inhale as you slowly bend your elbows. Lower yourself until your elbows are at a 90-degree angle.

5. Exhale and push back up through your hands to the start position. Control your body through the entire movement; don't let gravity do part of the work for you.

**Pro Tip:** To help reduce the possibility of pain, keep your arms in a neutral position, meaning your elbows stay tucked in close to your body and don't flare out during the exercise. Also, make sure you don't lower yourself where your elbows pass 90 degrees relative to your body.

### Straight-Leg Hamstring Bridge

The hamstrings are an often-neglected muscle group, yet they are one of the biggest muscle groups in the body. It is important to have strong hamstrings so we can perform our cardiovascular training and other exercises with a lowered injury risk.

Sets/Reps: 3 sets of 25-second holds.

1. Lie on your back with your legs fully extended, arms out 45 degrees at your side, and palms facing down.
2. Pushing down into your Achilles tendon/heels, lift your lower body and glutes off of the ground.
3. Lift as high as you can and squeeze your glutes to hold the position for 25 seconds.
4. Do your best to allow limited knee bend and keep your hips off of the ground.

**Pro Tip:** Try elevating your legs or try the exercise on one leg to increase difficulty.

### Bicep Curls

There's something to be said for enjoyment in exercise, and I find most people enjoy "working their arms." If you have dumbbells, paint cans, water jugs, soup cans, resistance bands, etc., find at least one of these items. It's time to curl!

Sets/Reps: 3 sets of 12 reps on each arm.

1. Stand up straight with your feet about hip-width apart.
2. Hold your object balanced in your hand/fingers with your palm facing away from you and your arm extended/relaxed.
3. Keeping a straight back and resisting movement at your shoulder joint, bend at your elbow and begin curling the weight toward your shoulder.
4. Make sure your elbow stays in a mostly fixed position, your arms stay tight to your torso, and

you're not using your back to help swing the weight upward.

5. Stop at about chest height, squeeze your bicep for about half a second, then slowly and with control lower back to the starting position and immediately go again.
6. Repeat 12 times on each side, then switch arms.

**Pro Tip:** Change the orientation of your wrist to hit different sections of your bicep muscle, making sure you monitor and avoid any pain you notice.

### *Core Hollow Body Hold*

This is another core exercise that can be done without excessive spinal movement and with limited equipment. The hollow body hold utilizes your own body's physics to create tension in your core.

Sets/Reps: 3 sets of 25-second holds.

1. Lie on your back with arms extended overhead and legs extended down.
2. Lift your upper body and lower body off of the ground to 45 degrees.
3. Your arms should remain straight without elbow bend, and your knees should remain straight without knee bend.
4. Focus on squeezing your core and breathing as you hold for 25 seconds.
5. Return to the starting position.

**Pro Tip:** Add a single arm press in the hollow body hold position to recruit even more core muscles.

*Wall Sit*

A wall sit is a great way to build lower-body strength while also teaching good, upright posture. Remember to keep breathing as you hold this position.

Sets/Reps: 3 sets of 45-second holds (feel free to change the time based on your abilities).

1. Find a sturdy/flat service like a concrete wall and position yourself about two feet away from said wall.
2. Place your entire back/shoulders and head against the wall while keeping your feet about two feet away.
3. Keeping contact on the wall with your head, back, and shoulders, slowly descend into a squat position, letting your knees bend until your quads (thighs) are parallel with the ground.
4. Hold this 90-degree position for the time of your choosing based on your current fitness level.

**Pro Tip:** Increase duration over time or add weight to your lap to increase difficulty to allow for continued progress.

---

## Week 1, Day 4: Cardiovascular Training/Flexibility

*Intervals*

It's important that your heart works in various heart rate zones so that like your other muscles, it can get stronger and more efficient. The second day of cardio calls for a

172 | APPENDIX A

more interval-based approach where your heart rate will rise to higher levels than the first day, followed by "active rest" periods.

**Sets/Reps: 10 rounds of 20 seconds of work and 2 minutes of rest.**

Try starting with a 1:6 work-to-rest ratio, meaning for every one second of work, you are going to rest for six seconds to ensure enough recovery between sets for optimal performance. Choose whatever form of cardio you enjoy and your body allows, whether that be cycling on a bicycle or stationary bike, running outside or on a treadmill, using an elliptical, etc. The piece of equipment you choose is not a huge factor; however, pushing yourself to the appropriate levels of intensity is crucial to the effectiveness of this style of training. Make sure you do a light, dynamic warm-up before you start. I often recommend using the cardio modality of your choice and doing less intense warm-up sets (1–3 sets total) at about 50 percent of your max intensity to prepare and prime your body for the more intense sets. Based on your current level of fitness, push yourself to about 60–70 percent for beginners and 70–80 percent for the well-trained folks during the "work" phase of the interval. During your "rest" interval, it's important that you do not completely stop, as this can cause muscles to get tight due in part to a buildup of lactic acid from the intensity. Participate in active rest, in which you slow down to about 10–20 percent of max speed on whatever you're doing. For example, if you're sprinting, slow down to a walk, or if you're cycling, slow down to a slow pedal. Repeat 6–10 times.

**Pro Tip:** If you have a device to measure your heart rate, take note of how hard you push yourself and how fast your heart rate recovers (on your smart devices, this can be a measure of heart rate variability).

Follow your aerobic workout with a couple of the stretches you learned on Day 2:

1.  Supine active hamstring stretch
2.  Superman stretch

How do we progress from week to week?

---

## Weeks 2–4: Resistance Training/Core/Balance

Your body adapts best when appropriate levels of volume, intensity, and resistance are practiced consistently over time. In other words, it's much smarter to stick with a training program for four, eight, or even twelve or more weeks, depending on conditions, rather than trying to do something new every time you work out.

It also gives you time to master certain exercises and "own" movements until you're ready to progress to the next level/phase of training. With that being said, make sure you give yourself the time to completely understand the exercises laid out for you and perform them with the proper form and level of difficulty.

Since this program is four weeks long, I'm going to explain how to progress yourself over the next three weeks until all four weeks are completed.

For your resistance training days, pick two exercises per workout to increase by one set. For example, say Week 1, Day 1 you chose step-ups and standing curl to overhead presses; Week 2, Day 2 would now have four sets of those exercises instead of three. Do the same for the following two weeks, making sure to disperse the volume you add. Keep in mind you shouldn't have more than five sets of one exercise. Also, try to add 2.5 to 10 percent of the load you did from week to week. For example, if you were able to do horizontal rows with ten pounds, try adding one to four pounds on Week 2. For body weight exercises, try adding one or two reps week to week or slow down the tempo by an extra one to two seconds. By Week 4, you should build up to weights with which you can only perform a few extra reps beyond the rep-range protocol with good form.

On the two separate cardiovascular days, your progression techniques will center around time, distance, and intensity. On your aerobic, a.k.a. lighter intensity, day, I recommend trying to add an additional five to ten minutes to your chosen exercise. For example, if you walked for thirty minutes Week 1, try to walk thirty-five or forty minutes Week 2.

# Heart-Healthy Menu, Dietary Analysis, Sample Grocery List

## Heart-Healthy Menu

An asterisk indicates an item that has a recipe in this appendix following the menu section.

*Week One*

**MONDAY**

BREAKFAST

*Egg white scramble*
- 2 scrambled eggs (with yolks separated out), 2 slices of whole-grain bread (100% whole wheat, or rye), $1/2$ cup cooked spinach, $1/4$ cup low-fat shredded cheese.

## LUNCH

*Sun-dried tomato spinach wrap*
- 1 tortilla wrap, spread 2 tbsp. red pepper hummus, a handful of spinach, tomatoes, red onions, sun-dried tomatoes, and sliced cucumbers.

## SNACK

- 1 whole bell pepper (any color) sliced; 2 tbsp. hummus or guacamole.

## DINNER

*Pan-seared salmon with citrus vinegar glaze and green beans\**
- 1 serving.

## TUESDAY

## BREAKFAST

*Grilled peanut butter and strawberry sandwich*
- 1 sandwich with whole-grain bread; 2 tbsp. all-natural nut butter (peanut, almond, sunflower seed); $1/2$ cup sliced strawberries (or other berry variety). Grill on medium-high heat in cooking pan 2–3 minutes each side.

## LUNCH

*Avocado egg salad on whole-grain bread*
- $1/2$ avocado, 2 boiled eggs, salt, pepper, garlic powder, $1/4$ onion mixed and served on whole-grain bread with shredded arugula/spinach mix.

## SNACK

- 2 oz. trail mix with nuts, seeds, and dried fruit; 1 cup blueberries.

## DINNER

*Grilled flatbread veggie pizza**
- 1 serving.
- 1 cup arugula/spinach mix salad with handful croutons and 1 tbsp. choice of dressing.

# WEDNESDAY

## BREAKFAST

- Low-fat plain Greek yogurt (6 oz.), 1 cup raspberries, 2 tbsp. chopped walnuts or granola.

## LUNCH

*Veggie pizza salad*
- 1 slice of veggie pizza, 1 cup of chopped kale, 1 cup of chopped red cabbage, 1/2 cucumber, sliced. 2 tbsp. of salad dressing of choice. Slice pizza into crouton-size pieces and place on salad.

## SNACK

- 1 cup sliced strawberries, 1 handful almonds.

## DINNER

*Tuna salad on bib lettuce*
- 2 pouches or cans (drained) white tuna, 1/2 red onion,

1 stalk of celery, pepper, $1/2$ avocado, 1 tbsp. mayo, garlic powder, and relish (optional). Mix together and serve on bib lettuce. Serve with 1 cup of fruit salad (mango, pineapple, kiwi, and dark cherries).

## THURSDAY

### BREAKFAST

*Oats with apples and blueberries*
- Mix together $1/2$ cup cooked oats, $1/2$ cup unsweetened almond milk, $1/2$ cup chopped apple, $1/4$ cup blueberries (frozen or fresh), $1/4$ cup chopped walnuts or slivered almonds, 1 tsp. cinnamon, and 1 tsp. vanilla extract.

### LUNCH

*Tuna whole-grain pita*
- Stuff 1 whole-grain pita with chopped onions, celery, shredded carrots, 1 packet of tuna, $1/2$ cup spinach leaves, and choice of dressing or mayo.

### SNACK

- 1 cup fruit salad (mango, pineapple, kiwi, and cherries), 1 handful pistachios.

### DINNER

*Grilled Asian garlic steak skewers\**
- 1 serving; serve with green salad.

## FRIDAY

### BREAKFAST

*Two-egg omelet with veggies*
- Cook $1/2$ cup spinach and mushrooms with olive oil. Add 2 scrambled eggs on top of veggies and cook on medium heat. Flip and add 1 oz. cheddar cheese. Fold into omelet.

### LUNCH

*PB & J with sliced strawberries and bananas*
- 2 slices whole-grain bread, 2 tbsp. peanut butter, 1 tbsp. natural jam, sliced strawberries and bananas on sandwich.

### SNACK

- 3 cups air-popped popcorn.

### DINNER

*Grilled veggie sandwich\**
- Serve with garden salad; 1 sandwich.

## SATURDAY

### BREAKFAST

*Heart-healthy smoothie*
- 1 cup blueberries, 1 cup low-fat milk, 2 tbsp. ground flax, hemp or chia seed, 2 tbsp. peanut butter, ice (add spinach or kale for extra vitamins and minerals).

## LUNCH

*Lettuce wrap*
- 4 slices low-sodium roast turkey or ham, 1 slice low-fat cheese, shredded carrots, 1 tbsp. hummus, wrapped in lettuce; 6 whole-grain crackers. Serve with $1/2$ veggie sandwich.

## SNACK

- 1 large apple with 2 tbsp. all-natural nut butter (peanut, almond, sunflower seed).

## DINNER

*Seared scallops with butternut squash\**
- 1 serving.

# SUNDAY

## BREAKFAST

- Low-fat plain Greek yogurt (6 oz.), 1 cup blackberries, 2 tbsp. chopped walnuts or granola.

## LUNCH

- 1 cup low-fat cottage cheese, 1 cup blueberries, 1 handful almonds.

## SNACK

- 1 cup fruit salad (mango, pineapple, kiwi, and cherries), 1 handful almonds.

## DINNER

*Black bean quesadilla**
* 1 serving.

*Week Two*

# MONDAY

## BREAKFAST

* 1 cup oatmeal (cooked in low-fat milk), 1 cup blueberries.

## LUNCH

* 1 cup tossed salad mix—with any non-starchy vegetables (i.e., string beans, broccoli, cabbage, spinach).
  Add 2 hardboiled eggs, dress with 1 tbsp. vinegar and
  olive oil; 1 cup melon.

## SNACK

* 20 baby carrots with 2 tbsp. hummus or 2 tbsp.
  guacamole.

## DINNER

*Broiled cod with pesto tomatoes**
* 1 serving.

# TUESDAY

## BREAKFAST

* 1 1/4 cup whole-grain cereal, 1 cup low-fat milk, 1 cup
  berries, 1 handful chopped almonds.

## LUNCH

- 1 whole wheat pita stuffed with 1 cup shredded romaine lettuce, $^1/_2$ cup sliced tomatoes, $^1/_4$ cup sliced cucumbers, 2 tbsp. crumbled feta cheese, and 1 tbsp. flaxseed oil and vinegar; 1 kiwi or choice of fruit.

## SNACK

- Medium orange, 1 handful nuts.

## DINNER

*Grilled salmon (6 oz.)\**
- Grill on high 8 minutes per side, season with olive oil, salt, pepper, lemon/lime, and garlic powder; 1 cup steamed broccoli; 1 medium baked sweet potato. Top with cinnamon and a dollop of low-fat plain Greek yogurt.

## WEDNESDAY

### BREAKFAST

- 2 whole grain waffles with 2 tbsp. peanut or almond butter; 1 cup blueberries; 6 oz. vanilla Greek yogurt.

### LUNCH

*Salmon salad*
- 1 salmon pouch, $^1/_2$ cup chickpeas (if using canned, make sure to rinse), $^1/_2$ cup chopped red onion, $^1/_2$ cup chopped red bell pepper; 2 cups romaine lettuce; dress with 1 tbsp. extra virgin olive oil and 2 tbsp. red-wine vinegar.

## SNACK

- 1 apple, 1 cheese stick or 1 oz. fresh mozzarella cheese.

## DINNER

*Strawberry goat cheese salad with grilled chicken\**
- 2 tbsp. choice of dressing; 1 serving.

# THURSDAY

## BREAKFAST

*Green smoothie bowl\**
- 1 serving.

## LUNCH

*Edamame, feta, tomato salad*
- 1 cup shelled edamame, 1 handful feta cheese, 1 cup tomatoes, 1/4 diced red onion, 1 chopped apple, 2 tbsp. choice of dressing.

## SNACK

- 1 cup low-fat cottage cheese, 1 cup raspberries, 1 handful chopped almonds.

## DINNER

*Chicken and vegetable stir-fry\**
- 1 serving.

## FRIDAY

### BREAKFAST

*Egg omelet with peppers, onions, and mushrooms*
- 2 eggs, 2 slices whole grain bread, 1 cup peppers, onions, mushrooms, 1 tbsp. shredded low-fat cheese.

### LUNCH

*Brown rice bowl*
- $2/3$ cup brown rice, 1 piece (4 oz.) premade chicken, 1 cup mixed vegetables (broccoli, peppers, carrots).

### SNACK

- 1 cup sliced strawberries, 1 handful walnuts.

### DINNER

*Grilled turkey veggie burgers\**
- Serve with roasted glazed carrots\*; 1 serving.

## SATURDAY

### BREAKFAST

*Oats and fruit*
- $1/2$ cup cooked oatmeal, $1/2$ diced apple or pear, 2 tbsp. chopped nuts, $1/2$ cup low-fat milk.

### LUNCH

- 1 cup cottage cheese, $1/2$ cup sliced apple, $1/4$ cup sunflower seeds.

## SNACK

- 2 handfuls almonds, 1 banana.

## DINNER

*Weeknight Mediterranean pasta\**
- 1 serving.

# SUNDAY

## BREAKFAST

- 1 boiled egg, 1 cup low-fat milk, 1 cup high-fiber cereal with 1 sliced banana on top.

## LUNCH

*Yogurt bowl*
- 1 cup nonfat Greek yogurt, $1/2$ tablespoon flaxseed meal, $1/2$ tablespoon chia seeds, 1 tablespoon almond butter, 1 cup assorted fresh fruit (sliced strawberries and bananas, nectarine wedges, blueberries, etc.), 2 tbsp. granola, drizzle of honey, sprinkle of coconut flakes.

## SNACK

- $1/4$ cup hummus; 1 medium red bell pepper, sliced; 3 medium carrots, sliced.

## DINNER

*Roasted halibut with herb salad\**
- 1 serving.

## *Week Three*

## MONDAY

### BREAKFAST

*Whole-grain toast with pears and honey*
- 1 slice whole-grain toast topped with 2 tbsp. almond butter, 1 sliced pear, 2 tsp. honey, 1 orange zest, 2 tbsp. unsalted sliced almonds.

### LUNCH

*Mediterranean bistro box*
- $^1/_2$ sliced cucumber, $^1/_4$ cup hummus, 2 tbsp. olives, 1 handful feta cheese, 1 whole wheat pita cut into four pieces.

### SNACK

- 3 tbsp. unsalted almonds, 2 medium carrots.

### DINNER

*Easy shrimp and vegetable skillet\**
- 1 serving.

## TUESDAY

### BREAKFAST

- 2 scrambled eggs, 2 slices whole-grain bread. Add feta (1 handful), chopped tomatoes, and spinach or mixed veggies, $^1/_3$ avocado.

## LUNCH

*Goat cheese beet salad*
- 2 cups spring mix greens, topped with 1 spoonful crumbled goat cheese, $1/2$ cup beets, $1/4$ cup sunflower seeds, $1/4$ cup dried cherries, and 2 tbsp. raspberry vinaigrette.

## SNACK

- 1 medium orange, 1 cheese stick or fresh mozzarella.

## DINNER

*Grilled chicken with spaghetti squash\**
- 1 serving.

# WEDNESDAY

## BREAKFAST

- Low-fat plain Greek yogurt (6 oz.), $3/4$ cup blueberries, 1 handful almonds or 2 tbsp. ground flaxseed meal.

## LUNCH

- (Recommend using a three-compartment container.)
- Large section: raw broccoli and carrots.
- Small section: almonds.
- Small section: dried fruit.

## SNACK

- 1 handful mixed nuts, unsalted; 1 cup fresh strawberries and blueberries.

## DINNER

*Fish tacos*
- (Serving size 2 tacos.) Bake cod (6 oz.) at 400 degrees for 13–15 minutes. Season cod with 2 tbsp. olive oil, garlic, pepper, paprika, and lemon. Place 3 oz. in each whole corn tortilla wrap. Add chopped tomatoes, sautéed peppers and onions. Add ¼ avocado, shredded lettuce, and 1 handful low-fat shredded cheese.

## THURSDAY

### BREAKFAST

*Avocado toast with optional smoked salmon\**

### LUNCH

*Make-ahead tuna baguette sandwich*
- Slice open 6" baguette. Combine 1 tuna packet in oil, olives, garlic powder, and 2 tsp. red wine vinegar. Add sliced tomatoes, red onion, 1 sliced hard-boiled egg, and fresh basil leaves.

### SNACK

- 2 handfuls whole-grain crackers with hummus on top; 1 cup sliced carrots and peppers.

### DINNER

*Easy Greek salad\**
- 2 cups.

## FRIDAY

### BREAKFAST

- 1 cup plain oatmeal (regular or instant), ¾ cup sliced berries, ¼ cup chopped walnuts or slivered almonds.

### LUNCH

*Greek salad*
- 2 cups of leftovers from previous day.

### SNACK

- ½ cup roasted edamame (store-bought or home-made), 1 banana.

### DINNER

*Honey garlic glazed salmon\**
- 1 serving. Serve with 1 cup roasted asparagus.

## SATURDAY

### BREAKFAST

- 1 whole-grain English muffin with 1 tbsp. peanut butter, 1 cup blueberries, 1 cup low-fat milk.

## LUNCH

*Avocado garden sandwich*
- 2 slices whole-grain bread, 1 avocado, lettuce, arugula, tomatoes, red onion, 1 slice provolone cheese, and 1 tsp. mayo.

## SNACK

- Three 6" fruit skewers dipped in Greek yogurt (pineapple, strawberry, and mango).

## DINNER

*Baked chicken and veggies\**
- 1 serving.

## SUNDAY

## BREAKFAST

- 1 whole-grain bread sandwich thin (at least 3 grams of fiber), or whole-grain English muffin, 2 tbsp. all-natural nut butter (peanut, almond, sunflower seed), 1/2 cup sliced strawberries (or other berry variety).

## LUNCH

*Baked chicken salad*
- (Leftovers.) 4 oz. baked premade chicken over 2 cups spinach, 1 handful fresh mozzarella, olives, tomatoes, cucumber, and 1/4 avocado. Dress with 3 tbsp. flaxseed oil vinaigrette\* or EVOO vinaigrette\*.

## SNACK

*Peanut butter energy balls*
- 2 cups rolled oats, 1 cup natural peanut butter or other nut butter, $1/2$ cup honey, $1/4$ cup mini chocolate chips, $1/4$ cup unsweetened shredded coconut. Use tablespoon to measure each ball. Serving size 2 balls.

## DINNER

*Veggie pasta primavera\**
- 1 serving.

*Week Four*

# MONDAY

## BREAKFAST

*French toast*
- 2 slices whole-grain bread. Mix 1 egg, $1/4$ cup unsweetened almond milk or cow's milk, 1 tsp. vanilla, 1 tsp. cinnamon. (Dip bread into batter, then cook in pan coated with olive oil.)

## LUNCH

- (Recommend using a three-compartment container.)
- Large section: sliced apples.
- Small section: cottage cheese.
- Small section: halved walnuts.

## SNACK

- 1 oz. low-sodium turkey breast and 1 oz. cheese, 5–6 whole-grain crackers, 1 cup blueberries.

## DINNER

*Easy one-pan roasted shrimp and veggies\**
- 1 serving.

# TUESDAY

## BREAKFAST

- 1 cup low-fat cottage cheese, $1/2$ cup sliced apple, 2 tbsp. chopped almonds.

## LUNCH

*Salmon salad pita*
- Mix together 2 oz. canned salmon, 1 tbsp. low-fat mayo, squeeze of lemon, pepper, paprika, cumin. Add shredded lettuce and salmon into pita. Serve with orange slices and celery sticks.

## SNACK

- For a smoothie, blend 6 oz. Greek yogurt, 6 oz. 100% fruit juice, $1/2$ banana, $1/2$ mango, $1/2$ cup frozen strawberries; $1/2$ oz. pistachios.

## DINNER

*20-minute chicken tacos*
- Serve with veggies. Sauté 2 cups carrots, scallions, zucchini, and peppers with 1 tbsp. olive oil. Serving size 2 tacos.

## WEDNESDAY

### BREAKFAST

- For a smoothie, blend 1 banana, 1 cup low-fat milk, 2 tbsp. ground flax, hemp or chia seeds, 2 tbsp. peanut butter, ice. (Add spinach/kale for extra vitamins and minerals.)

### LUNCH

*Chicken chow mein salad*
- 2 cups salad greens or spinach, 2 oz. rotisserie or pre-made chicken, 1/2 cup red cabbage, 1 tbsp. pecans, 1 tbsp. cranberries, 2 tbsp. low-sodium ginger and soy dressing.

### SNACK

- 1 apple (sliced), with 2 tbsp. peanut butter. Top with 1/4 cup mixture of dried cherries, blueberries, and crushed almonds.

### DINNER

*Marinated veggie beef kebabs**
- 1 serving.

## THURSDAY

### BREAKFAST

- 1/2 cup low-sugar granola, low-fat or nonfat Greek yogurt (6 oz.), 1 cup berries.

## LUNCH

- Leftover beef kebab over 2 cups mixed greens. Add mixed veggies (cucumber, tomato, and carrots), 2 tbsp. choice of dressing.

## SNACK

- 2 oz. trail mix with nuts, seeds, and dried fruit, 1 cup strawberries, 1 cup low-fat milk.

## DINNER

*Baked turkey quinoa spinach meatballs\**
- 1 serving. Serve with $1/2$ cup whole-grain rice.

# FRIDAY

## BREAKFAST

*Egg sandwich*
- Low-sodium turkey (2 slices), 2 scrambled eggs, 1 whole-grain English muffin or 1 whole-grain sandwich thin, 1 tbsp. shredded low-fat cheddar, 2 slices medium tomato.

## LUNCH

*Egg roll in a bowl*
- $1/2$ cup ground premade turkey on top of $1/2$ cup whole-grain rice. Add 1 cup premade shredded veggies (kale, cabbage and carrots). Add garlic (fresh or powder), ginger (fresh or power), 1 tbsp. low-sodium soy sauce, and 2 tbsp. rice vinegar.

## SNACK

- 1 cup low-fat cottage cheese, $1/2$ cup blackberries.

## DINNER

*Spicy salmon bowl\**
- 1 serving.

# SATURDAY

## BREAKFAST

- 2 scrambled eggs, 2 slices whole-grain bread (100% whole wheat or rye), $1/2$ cup cooked spinach, $1/4$ cup low-fat shredded cheese.

## LUNCH

- 1 cup chopped carrots, cauliflower, and green peppers with 2 tbsp. hummus and leftover spicy salmon bowl ($1/2$–1 serving).

## SNACK

- For a smoothie, blend $1/2$ cup ice, 6 oz. plain Greek yogurt, $1/2$ banana, $1/2$ mango, $1/2$ cup frozen strawberries, and $1/4$ cup orange juice. Add liquid (water) to reach desired consistency.

## DINNER

*Mediterranean pasta salad\**
- 1 serving. Serve with 2 oz. whole-grain bread or baguette.

## SUNDAY

### BREAKFAST

*Apple oatmeal*
- 1 cup oatmeal (cooked in milk), 1 cup diced apple, 1 tsp. cinnamon, 2 tbsp. chopped walnuts.

### LUNCH

- 1 cup leftover Mediterranean pasta salad over 2 cups mixed greens, 2 tbsp. choice of dressing.

### SNACK

- 1 cup carrot and celery sticks, 2 tbsp. peanut butter, 1/2 cup fresh blackberries or raspberries.

### DINNER

*Low-sodium turkey chili\**
- 1 serving.

---

## Week One Recipes

### PAN-SEARED SALMON WITH CITRUS VINEGAR GLAZE AND GREEN BEANS

*Ingredients*

4 (6 oz.) portions salmon fillets

Extra virgin olive oil, for brushing fish

Salt and pepper

1/2 cup dry white wine

1/2 cup balsamic vinegar

2 tbsp. orange juice (a splash)

2 tsp. lemon juice

2 tbsp. brown sugar

1 lb. green beans, trimmed

Orange slices or lemon rind

### Directions (Servings: 4)

1. Preheat a cast iron pan or heavy-bottomed skillet over medium high heat. Brush salmon fillets with oil. Season with salt and pepper. Cook salmon until just cooked through, about three minutes on each side.
2. While salmon cooks, bring wine, vinegar, citrus juices, and brown sugar to a boil over high heat. Reduce glaze three or four minutes, until thickened. Remove from heat. Stir in $1/2$ tsp. coarse black pepper.
3. In a second skillet, bring $1/2$" water to a boil with green beans and pieces of orange and/or lemon rind. Cover the green beans and cook three or four minutes. Drain beans and toss with a drizzle of oil (optional) and season with salt and pepper.
4. Drizzle glaze over salmon fillets and serve with citrus green beans.

## GRILLED FLATBREAD VEGGIE PIZZA

### Ingredients

1 tbsp. olive oil

$1/2$ lb. sliced baby Portobello mushrooms

1 large green pepper, julienned

4 cups fresh baby spinach (about 4 oz.)

$1/4$ tsp. salt

$1/8$ tsp. pepper

2 naan flatbreads or 4 whole pita breads

2 tbsp. olive oil

$1/4$ cup prepared pesto

2 plum tomatoes, sliced

2 cups shredded part-skim mozzarella cheese

*Directions (Servings: 4)*

1. In a large skillet, heat olive oil over medium-high heat. Add mushrooms and green pepper; cook and stir five to seven minutes or until tender. Add spinach, salt and pepper; cook and stir two to three minutes or until spinach is wilted.
2. Brush both sides of flatbreads with oil. Grill flatbreads, covered, over medium heat two to three minutes on one side or until lightly browned.
3. Remove from grill. Spread grilled sides with pesto; top with vegetable mixture, tomatoes, and cheese. Return to grill; cook, covered, two to three minutes longer or until cheese is melted.
4. Cut pizzas in half before serving.

## GRILLED ASIAN GARLIC STEAK SKEWERS

*Ingredients*

1 1/2 lbs. top sirloin steak
1 red onion
2/3 cup low sodium soy sauce
6 garlic cloves, minced
1/4 cup sesame oil
1/2 cup vegetable oil

1/3 cup sugar
1 tbsp. grated ginger
2 tbsp. sesame seeds
Sliced green onions for garnish
Skewers

*Directions (Servings: 6)*

1. Cut steak into 1" cubes. Cut red onion into large chunks and set aside.
2. In a large bowl, whisk together soy sauce, garlic, sesame oil, vegetable oil, sugar, ginger, and sesame seeds. Add steak and toss to coat in marinade. Marinate for three hours or overnight.

3. Preheat grill to medium-high heat. Thread meat and red onion onto skewers. Grill for eight to ten minutes until meat is done to desired liking.

## GRILLED VEGGIE SANDWICH

*Ingredients*

1 medium zucchini, thinly sliced lengthwise into ribbons

1 medium sweet red pepper, quartered

1 small red onion, cut into 1/2" slices

1/4 cup prepared Italian salad dressing

1 loaf ciabatta bread (14

oz.), split

2 tbsp. olive oil

1/4 cup reduced-fat mayonnaise

1 tbsp. lemon juice

2 tsp. grated lemon zest

1 tsp. minced garlic

1/2 cup crumbled feta cheese

*Directions (Servings: 4)*

1. In a bowl or shallow dish, combine zucchini, pepper, onion, and salad dressing. Cover and turn to coat; refrigerate for at least one hour. Drain and discard marinade.

2. Brush cut sides of bread with oil; set aside. Place vegetables on grill rack. Grill, covered, over medium heat for four to five minutes on each side or until crisp-tender. Remove and keep warm. Grill bread, oil side down, over medium heat for thirty to sixty seconds or until toasted. (If no grill, can roast in oven. Place veggies on baking sheet and roast for thirty minutes at 400° F).

3. In a small bowl, combine mayonnaise, lemon juice, zest, and garlic. Spread over cut side of bread bottom; sprinkle with cheese. Top with vegetables and remaining bread. Cut into four slices.

## SEARED SCALLOPS WITH BUTTERNUT SQUASH

*Ingredients*

2 lbs. butternut squash; peeled, seeded, and cut into 1" chunks

1 tbsp. half-and-half

2 tbsp. unsalted butter

2 tbsp. olive oil

Salt and pepper

$1/8$ teaspoon cayenne

pepper

1 $1/2$ lbs. sea scallops; tendons removed

2 tbsp. vegetable oil

1 shallot; minced

8 whole sage leaves

1 tbsp. lemon juice

*Directions (Servings: 4)*

1. Place squash in microwave-safe bowl, cover, and microwave until tender, eight to twelve minutes, stirring squash halfway through. Drain, then transfer squash to food processor. Add half-and-half, 1 tbsp. olive oil, $1/2$ tsp. salt, and cayenne, and process until smooth. Transfer to bowl and cover to keep warm.

2. Pat scallops dry with paper towels and season with salt and pepper. Heat 1 tbsp. oil in large nonstick skillet over high heat until just smoking. Add half of scallops and cook, without moving them, until well browned, one-and-a-half to two minutes. Turn scallops and cook until sides are firm and opaque, thirty

to ninety seconds. Transfer scallops to plate and tent loosely with foil. Wipe out skillet with paper towels and repeat with remaining oil and scallops. Transfer to plate with first batch.

3. Heat remaining butter over medium heat, swirling skillet constantly, until butter has nutty aroma, about one minute. Add shallot, minced sage, and sage leaves, and cook until fragrant, about one minute. Off heat, stir in lemon juice and season with salt and pepper. Pour sauce over scallops and serve with butternut squash.

## BLACK BEAN QUESADILLA

*Ingredients*

2 whole wheat tortillas

2 oz. reduced fat Monterey Jack cheese, shredded ($1/2$ cup)

$1/2$ cup canned black beans, drained

$1/4$ cup canned diced green chiles

$1/2$ tsp. olive oil

*Directions (Servings: 2)*

1. Spread cheese, beans, and chiles on one tortilla and top with another.
2. Heat oil in a fry pan over medium heat and add the quesadilla.
3. Cook for about seven minutes, turning over halfway through.
4. Remove to a plate and cut into serving wedges.

## Week Two Recipes

### BROILED COD WITH PESTO TOMATOES

*Ingredients*

1 large ripe tomato, cored and sliced very thinly (about 1/8")

Kosher salt and freshly ground black pepper

2 tbsp. extra virgin olive oil

1 1/2 cups panko bread crumbs

1 small clove garlic, minced

1–1 1/2 lb. cod or haddock, rinsed, patted dry, and cut into four even portions

2/3 cup premade basil pesto

*Directions (Servings: 4)*

1. Heat oven to 450° F.
2. Spread tomato slices on a large plate and season with a pinch of salt and a few grinds of black pepper.
3. Heat a large sauté pan over medium heat for one minute. Pour in olive oil, add breadcrumbs, and season with a pinch of salt. Cook, stirring, until breadcrumbs start to turn a light golden brown, about four minutes. Add garlic and continue to cook, stirring, for another minute. Transfer to a bowl.
4. Set fish on a large-rimmed baking sheet lined with foil. Season with salt and pepper. Divide pesto evenly over fish and top each with two or three tomato slices and breadcrumbs. Roast until fish is opaque on the sides and starts to flake, about ten minutes. Serve immediately.

## STRAWBERRY GOAT CHEESE SALAD WITH GRILLED CHICKEN

*Ingredients*

4 cups baby arugula

4 cups baby spring green mix

1 cup farro, cooked according to package directions

1 cup strawberries, hulled and halved

1/2 cup blueberries

4 oz. goat cheese, crumbled

1/4 cup almonds, roughly chopped

Kosher salt and ground black pepper, to season

### For the grilled herb chicken:

*Ingredients*

Optional: 1 tbsp. olive oil

1 lb. boneless, skinless chicken breasts

1 tsp. kosher salt

1 tsp. ground black

pepper

1 tsp. fresh thyme, finely chopped

1 tsp. fresh rosemary, finely chopped

*Directions (Servings: 4)*

1. Bring large pot of salted water to a boil and cook the farro according to package directions. I recommend finding a "quick-cook" farro, which will take about ten to fifteen minutes to cook. Once cooked to al dente, drain farro and rinse with cool water. Set aside or store in an airtight container in the refrigerator for up to one week. As farro cooks, get started on prepping the rest of the salad.

2. As farro cooks, grill chicken. Preheat grill or grill pan

to medium-high heat. If using a grill pan, add in 1 tbsp. of olive oil. Season both sides of chicken breasts with salt, pepper, thyme, and rosemary. Once grill is nice and hot, place chicken on grates. Grill chicken for six to eight minutes per side, or until chicken has beautifully charred grill marks and is cooked all the way through. Transfer chicken to a plate to rest for a few minutes before slicing it into bite-sized pieces.

3. Assemble strawberry salad: In a large serving dish or bowl, arrange arugula and spring green mix. Top with strawberries, blueberries, farro, crumbled goat cheese, and chopped almonds. Arrange sliced grilled chicken over top.

## GREEN SMOOTHIE BOWL

**Smoothie:**

*Ingredients*

- 1/4 ripe avocado
- 2 medium ripe bananas (previously sliced and frozen)
- 1 cup fresh or frozen mixed berries
- 2 large handfuls spinach
- 1 small handful kale
- 1 1/2–2 cups unsweetened non-dairy milk
- 1 tbsp. flaxseed meal
- 2 tbsp. salted creamy almond or peanut butter (optional)

**Toppings (optional):**

*Ingredients*

- Granola
- Raw or roasted nuts (almonds, pecans, walnuts, etc.)
- Shredded unsweetened coconut
- Fresh berries

*Directions (Servings: 2)*

1. Add all smoothie ingredients to a blender and blend until creamy and smooth. Add more almond milk (or water) to thin.

## CHICKEN AND VEGETABLE STIR-FRY

*Ingredients*

1 lb. boneless, skinless chicken breasts cut into 1" cubes

Salt and pepper to taste

2 tbsp. olive oil divided

2 cups broccoli florets

1/2 yellow bell pepper cut into 1" pieces

1/2 red bell pepper cut into 1" pieces

1/2 cup baby carrots sliced

2 tsp. minced ginger

2 garlic cloves, minced

### Stir-Fry Sauce
*Ingredients*

1 tbsp. corn starch

2 tbsp. cold water

1/4 cup low sodium chicken broth

3 tbsp. low sodium soy sauce

1/4 cup honey

1 tbsp. toasted sesame oil

1/2 tsp. crushed red pepper flakes

*Directions (Servings: 4)*

1. In a medium bowl, whisk together corn starch and water. Add remaining ingredients (chicken broth, soy sauce, honey, and toasted sesame oil, red pepper flakes) and whisk to combine. Set aside.

2. Add 1 tbsp. of olive oil to a large skillet or wok and heat over medium-high heat.

3. Add chicken (in batches if necessary) and season with salt and pepper. Cook for three to five minutes or until cooked through. Remove from skillet.

4. Reduce heat to medium and add remaining table-spoon of oil to skillet.

5. Add broccoli, bell pepper, and carrots and cook, stir-ring occasionally, just until crisp tender. Add ginger and garlic and cook for an additional minute.

6. Add chicken back into skillet and stir to combine.

7. Whisk stir-fry sauce and pour over chicken and vege-tables and stir gently to combine.

8. Bring to a boil, stirring occasionally, and let boil for one minute.

9. Serve with rice and/or chow mein if desired.

## GRILLED TURKEY VEGGIE BURGERS

*Ingredients*

1 tbsp. extra virgin olive oil

1/2 cup finely diced onion

1/2 cup finely diced red bell pepper

Salt to taste

1 large garlic clove, green shoot removed, minced

2/3 cup finely grated carrot (1 large carrot)

1 1/4 lbs. lean ground turkey breast

1 tbsp. prepared barbecue sauce

1 tbsp. ketchup

Freshly ground pepper to taste

Canola oil for the skillet

Whole-grain hamburger buns

Condiments of your choice

*Directions (Servings: 6)*

1. Heat olive oil over medium heat in a medium skillet and add onion. Cook, stirring, until it begins to soften,

about three minutes, and add diced red pepper and a generous pinch of salt. Cook, stirring often, until vegetables are tender, about five minutes. Stir in garlic and grated carrot and cook, stirring, for another minute or two, until carrots have softened slightly and the mixture is fragrant. Remove from heat.

2. In a large bowl, mash ground turkey with a fork. Add about ³/₄ tsp. kosher salt if desired, and mix in barbecue sauce, ketchup, and freshly ground pepper to taste. Add sautéed vegetables and mix together well. Shape into six patties, about ³/₄" thick. Chill for one hour if possible to facilitate handling.

3. Heat a nonstick griddle or a large nonstick frying pan over medium-high heat and brush with a small amount of canola oil, or prepare a medium-hot grill. When you can feel heat when you hold your hand above it, cook patties for four minutes on each side. Serve on whole-grain buns, with condiments of your choice.

## ROASTED GLAZED CARROTS

### Ingredients

| | |
|---|---|
| 2 lbs. carrots, peeled | ¹/₂ tsp. salt |
| ¹/₄ cup brown sugar, loosely packed | ¹/₄ tsp. black pepper |
| 2 garlic cloves, minced | Parsley for garnish (optional) |
| 3 tbsp. olive oil | |

### Directions (Servings: 4)

1. Preheat oven to 400° F.
2. Cut carrot on diagonal lengths. Halve thicker end so they are all roughly the same width.

3. Toss in a bowl with sugar, garlic, oil, salt, and pepper. Pour onto tray, spread out.
4. Roast for twenty minutes. Toss, then roast ten more minutes until soft and caramelized on edges with plenty of glaze left on the tray.
5. Toss carrots in the glaze, sprinkle with parsley if using. Serve warm.

## WEEKNIGHT MEDITERRANEAN PASTA

*Ingredients*

1 lb. thin whole-grain spaghetti

1/2 cup extra virgin olive oil

4 garlic cloves, crushed

Salt (a pinch)

1 cup chopped fresh parsley

12 oz. grape tomatoes, halved

3 scallions (green onions), top trimmed, both whites and greens chopped

1 tsp. black pepper

6 oz. marinated artichoke hearts, drained

1/4 cup pitted olives, halved

1/4 cup crumbled feta cheese

10–15 fresh basil leaves, torn

Zest of 1 lemon

Crushed red pepper flakes, optional

*Directions (Servings: 4)*

1. Follow package instructions to cook thin spaghetti pasta to al dente.
2. When pasta is almost cooked, heat extra virgin olive oil in a large cast-iron skillet over medium heat. Lower heat and add garlic and a pinch of salt. Cook for ten seconds, stirring regularly. Stir in parsley, tomatoes,

and chopped scallions. Cook over low heat until just warmed through, about thirty seconds or so.

3. When pasta is ready, remove from heat, drain cooking water, and return to its cooking pot. Pour warmed olive oil sauce in and toss to coat thoroughly. Add black pepper and toss again to coat.

4. Add remaining ingredients and toss one more time. Serve immediately in pasta bowls, and if you like, top each with more basil leaves and feta. Enjoy!

## ROASTED HALIBUT WITH HERB SALAD

*Ingredients*

1 1/4 lbs. skinless halibut fillets
1/4 tsp. kosher salt
Ground black pepper
2 tbsp. olive oil
1 large shallot, very thinly sliced
1 1/2 cups fresh mixed

soft herb leaves (such as flat-leaf parsley, chervil, and a small amount of more powerfully flavored tarragon)
1 1/2 tbsp. fresh lemon juice

*Directions (Servings: 4)*

1. Preheat oven to 300° F. Season fish with salt and, if desired, pepper, and let stand twenty minutes. Toss fish with oil in a bowl to evenly coat, and place in a baking dish. Drizzle remaining oil from bowl over fish. Bake at 300° F; check doneness after fifteen minutes by pressing flesh gently with your thumb. If fish flakes apart, it is ready. If not, cook an additional three to five minutes and check again.

2. Rinse shallot under cold running water; pat dry.

Once fish is cooked, mix warm oil from the baking dish with shallot, herbs, and juice. Serve with fish.

---

## Week Three Recipes

### EASY SHRIMP AND VEGETABLE SKILLET

*Ingredients*

2 lbs. peeled and deveined shrimp

2 small zucchinis

2 small yellow squash

3 small bell peppers any color

4 tbsp. olive oil

1 tbsp. butter

2 garlic cloves, finely chopped

1 tbsp. paprika

$1/2$ tbsp. Cajun seasoning

Salt and pepper to taste

Fresh parsley to garnish

*Directions (Servings: 4)*

1. Cut vegetables into bite-sized pieces.
2. Place shrimp into a medium bowl and add Cajun seasoning, paprika, salt, and olive oil. Mix well.
3. Heat a large skillet over medium-high heat. Add shrimp and cook for about six to seven minutes, or until cooked through. Remove shrimp from skillet and set aside.
4. To same skillet, add garlic, butter, and vegetables. Season with salt and stir-fry for about ten minutes, or until the vegetables are tender.
5. Return shrimp to the skillet, stir well, and garnish with parsley. Serve.

## GRILLED CHICKEN WITH SPAGHETTI SQUASH

*Ingredients*

1 medium spaghetti
squash (4 lbs.)

1 can (14 1/2 ounces)
diced tomatoes,
undrained

2 tbsp. prepared pesto

1/2 tsp. garlic powder

1/2 tsp. Italian seasoning

1/4 cup dry breadcrumbs

1/4 cup shredded
parmesan cheese

1 lb. boneless skinless
chicken breasts, cut

into 1/2" cubes

1 tbsp. plus 1 tsp. olive
oil, divided

1/2 lb. sliced fresh
mushrooms

1 medium onion,
chopped

1 garlic clove, minced

1/2 cup low sodium
chicken broth

1/3 cup shredded cheddar
cheese

*Directions (Servings: 5)*

1. Place scored spaghetti squash onto the lined baking
   sheet. Roast in oven for about thirty-five to forty-five
   minutes, flipping over halfway through. It's done
   when skin pierces fairly easily with a knife. The knife
   should be able to go in pretty deep with very slight
   resistance.

2. Meanwhile, in a blender, combine tomatoes, pesto,
   garlic powder, and Italian seasoning. Cover and process until blended; set aside. In a small bowl, combine
   breadcrumbs and parmesan cheese; set aside.

3. In a large skillet, cook chicken in 1 tbsp. oil until no
   longer pink; remove and keep warm. In same skillet,
   sauté mushrooms and onion in remaining oil until
   tender. Add garlic; cook one minute longer. Stir in

broth, chicken, and reserved tomato mixture. Bring to a boil. Reduce heat; simmer, uncovered, for five minutes.

4. When squash is cool enough to handle, use a fork to separate strands. In a large ovenproof skillet, layer half of squash, chicken mixture, and reserved crumb mixture. Repeat layers.

5. Bake, uncovered, at 350° for fifteen minutes or until heated through. Sprinkle with cheddar cheese. Broil 3–4" from the heat for five to six minutes or until cheese is melted and golden brown.

## AVOCADO TOAST WITH SMOKED SALMON

*Ingredients*

1 slice country or sourdough bread, approximately 1/2" thick

Extra virgin olive oil

1 tbsp. goat cheese

1/2 medium avocado

2 slices tomato from a medium tomato

3 thin slices red onion, cut in rounds from a medium onion

3 pieces thinly sliced smoked salmon

Freshly squeezed lemon juice to taste, from 1/2 lemon

Kosher salt and freshly ground black pepper

*Directions (Servings: 1)*

1. Lightly brush bread with olive oil and toast to desired level of doneness. Spread goat cheese over surface. Top with avocado and mash with a fork to cover entire surface. Top with tomato, red onion, and smoked salmon. Add lemon juice and sprinkle with salt and pepper. Serve.

## EASY GREEK SALAD

### Ingredients

6 tbsp. extra virgin olive oil

2 tbsp. fresh lemon juice

1/2 tsp. chopped garlic

1 tsp. red wine vinegar

1/2 tsp. dried oregano or 1 tsp. chopped fresh oregano

1/2 tsp. dried dill or 1 tsp. chopped fresh dill

Salt and freshly ground black pepper

3 large plum tomatoes, seeded and coarsely chopped

3/4 cucumber, peeled, seeded, and coarsely chopped

1/2 red onion, chopped

1 bell pepper, seeded and coarsely chopped

1/2 cup pitted black olives (preferably brine-cured), coarsely chopped

Heaping 1/2 cup crumbled feta cheese

### Directions (Servings: 6)

1. Make dressing: Whisk olive oil, lemon juice, garlic, vinegar, oregano, and dill together until blended. Season to taste with salt and freshly ground black pepper.
2. Make salad: Combine tomatoes, cucumber, onion, bell pepper, olives in a bowl. Toss with dressing. Sprinkle with cheese and serve.

## HONEY GARLIC GLAZED SALMON

### Ingredients

1/3 cup honey

1/4 cup low sodium soy sauce

2 tbsp. lemon juice

1 tsp. red pepper flakes

3 tbsp. extra virgin olive oil, divided

4 salmon fillets (6 oz.

each), patted dry with
a paper towel

Kosher salt

Freshly ground black

pepper

3 cloves garlic, minced

1 lemon, sliced into
rounds

*Directions (Servings: 4)*

1. In a medium bowl, whisk together honey, soy sauce, lemon juice, and red pepper flakes.
2. In a large skillet over medium-high heat, heat two tbsp. oil. When oil is hot but not smoking, add salmon skin-side up and season with salt and pepper. Cook salmon until deeply golden, about six minutes, then flip over and add remaining tablespoon of oil.
3. Add garlic to skillet and cook until fragrant, one minute. Add honey mixture and sliced lemons and cook until sauce is reduced by about a third. Baste salmon with sauce.
4. Garnish with sliced lemon and serve.

## BAKED CHICKEN AND VEGGIES

*Ingredients*

2 large boneless, skinless
chicken breasts

1 red bell pepper

1 green bell pepper

1 yellow bell pepper

1/2 small red onion

1 medium zucchini

1 cup broccoli florets

1/2 cup grape tomatoes
sliced in half

2 tbsp. olive oil

1/2 tsp. salt

1/2 tsp. black pepper

2 tsp. Italian seasoning

*Directions (Servings: 4)*

1. Preheat oven to 475° F. Spray a large baking sheet with cooking spray.
2. Chop all veggies into large (around 1") pieces. On a separate plate or cutting board chop all chicken into large cubes.
3. Place chicken and veggies on prepared baking sheet. Add olive oil, salt, pepper, and Italian seasoning. Toss to combine.
4. Bake for twenty to twenty-five minutes or until veggies are charred and chicken is cooked through. Internal chicken temperature should be at least 165°.
5. Serve immediately and enjoy!

## VEGGIE PASTA PRIMAVERA

*Ingredients*

10 oz. dry penne pasta
1/4 cup olive oil
1/2 medium red onion, sliced
1 large carrot, peeled and sliced into matchsticks
2 cups broccoli florets, cut into matchsticks
1 medium red bell pepper, sliced into matchsticks
1 medium yellow squash, sliced into quarter portions

1 medium zucchini, sliced into quarter portions
3–4 garlic cloves, minced
1 heaping cup of grape tomatoes, halved through the length
2 tsp. dried Italian seasoning
1/2 cup pasta water
2 tbsp. fresh lemon juice
1/2 cup shredded parmesan, divided
2 tbsp. chopped fresh parsley

*Directions (Servings: 5)*

1. Bring a large pot of water to a boil. Cook penne pasta in salted water according to package directions, reserve $1/2$ cup pasta water before draining.
2. Meanwhile, heat olive oil in a deep 12" skillet over medium-high heat.
3. Add red onion and carrot and sauté for two minutes.
4. Add broccoli and bell pepper, then sauté for two minutes.
5. Add squash and zucchini, then sauté two to three minutes or until veggies have nearly softened.
6. Add garlic, tomatoes, and Italian seasoning and sauté two minutes longer.
7. Pour veggies into now empty pasta pot or serving bowl, add drained pasta, drizzle in lemon juice, season with a little more salt as needed, and toss while adding in pasta water to loosen as desired.
8. Toss in $1/4$ cup parmesan and parsley, then serve with remaining parmesan on top.

## FLAXSEED OIL VINAIGRETTE OR EXTRA VIRGIN OLIVE OIL VINAIGRETTE

### Flaxseed Oil Vinaigrette
*Ingredients*

$1/4$ cup lemon juice

$1/4$ cup flaxseed oil

$1/4$ cup white balsamic vinegar

1 tbsp. Dijon mustard

1 clove garlic, minced

Salt and pepper

## Extra Virgin Olive Oil Vinaigrette

*Ingredients*

3/4–1 cup extra virgin
olive oil, or any good-
tasting oil
1/4 cup good-tasting

vinegar or lemon juice
1/2 tsp. salt
1/8–1/4 tsp. black pepper

Optional extras (choose one or two to taste):

1 minced shallot, 1
minced or grated
garlic clove
1/2–1 tsp. grainy mustard

1–2 tbsp. minced herbs
1–2 tbsp. finely grated
cheese
1/2–1 tsp. honey

*Directions (Serving Size: 2–3 tbsp.)*

Flaxseed Oil Vinaigrette

1. Whisk together lemon juice, flaxseed oil, white balsamic vinegar, Dijon mustard, minced garlic, salt, and pepper.

Extra Virgin Olive Oil Vinaigrette

1. If using a bowl, use a fork or whisk to rapidly blend vinaigrette together. If using a jar, top with the lid and shake until vinaigrette is combined. If using a blender, blend until vinaigrette is thoroughly combined.

———

# Week Four Recipes

## EASY ONE-PAN ROASTED SHRIMP AND VEGGIES

*Ingredients*

1 lb. raw shrimp
2 cups broccoli florets

1 zucchini (cubed or
sliced)

½ onion (cubed or sliced)

1 bell pepper (cubed or sliced, any color)

1 medium carrot or potato, thinly sliced

2 tbsp. olive oil

1 tsp. salt

1 tsp. Italian seasoning

¼ tsp. paprika

¼ tsp. black pepper

### Directions (Servings: 4)

1. Preheat oven to 425°F for at least ten minutes. Line a large sheet pan with foil and set aside.
2. Place veggies in a large bowl and sprinkle with half seasoning mix and 1 tbsp. oil. In another bowl, combine shrimp, remaining seasoning mix (half), and 1 tbsp. oil; set shrimp aside.
3. Pour veggies onto sheet pan and bake for twelve to fifteen minutes or until lightly charred. Add shrimp and bake for five minutes or until pink and tender.

## TWENTY-MINUTE CHICKEN TACOS

### Ingredients

1 lb. boneless, skinless chicken thighs or chicken breasts

2 cloves garlic, minced

1 tbsp. lime juice

2 tbsp. olive oil

1 tbsp. cilantro

½ tsp. jalapeno

½ tsp. or onion powder

½ tsp. salt or to taste

¼ tsp. black pepper

8 small corn or flour tortillas

Pico de Gallo

½ cup finely chopped onion

½ cup finely chopped tomato

¼ cup finely chopped cilantro

1 finely chopped jalapeño, deseeded

1 tsp. lime juice

Pinch of salt and pepper to taste

*Directions (Servings: 8 tacos)*

1. Add chicken, garlic, olive oil, lime, and spices, to a large bowl or zip-seal bag and stir or shake to combine.
2. Heat a large pan to medium-high heat. Cook chicken six to seven minutes per side or until it is no longer pink and the internal temperature of 165° F. Remove from heat and cool for at least five minutes. Slice or chop into small cubes.
3. While chicken is cooking, combine chopped tomato, jalapeno, onion, cilantro, and lime juice in a small bowl. Char tortillas on the stovetop over flame until lightly charred (this step is optional).
4. Assemble tacos by placing about 1/4 cup of chicken into each tortilla. Top with a few tbsp. of the onion-tomato mixture and a drizzle of cilantro sauce.

## MARINATED VEGGIE BEEF KEBABS

### Marinade
*Ingredients*

1/4 cup olive oil
1/4 cup low sodium soy sauce
1 1/2 tbsp. fresh lemon juice
1 1/2 tbsp. red wine vinegar
2 1/2 tbsp. Worcestershire sauce
1 tbsp. honey
2 tsp. Dijon
1 tbsp. minced garlic
1 tsp. freshly ground black pepper

### Kebabs
*Ingredients*

1 3/4 lbs. sirloin steak          (look for thicker

steaks), cut into 1 ¼"
pieces

8 oz. button or cremini
mushrooms, halved
(unless small, in which
case keep whole)

3 bell peppers (1 red, 1
green, 1 yellow) cut
into 1 ¼" pieces

1 large red onion, diced

into chunks (about 1
¼")

1 tbsp. olive oil, plus
more for brushing grill
grates

Salt and freshly ground
black pepper

½ tsp. garlic powder

10 wooden skewer sticks

## Marinade

*Directions (Servings: 5)*

1. In a mixing bowl whisk together all marinade
   ingredients.

## Kebabs

*Directions (Servings: 5)*

1. Place steak into a gallon-size resealable bag. Pour
   marinade over steak, then seal bag while pressing out
   excess air and massage marinade over steak. Transfer
   to refrigerator and allow to marinate three to six
   hours.
2. Preheat a grill over medium-high heat to about 425°
   (partway through preheating clean grill grates if they
   aren't already clean).
3. With veggies on cutting board, drizzle with oil and
   lightly toss to coat.
4. Sprinkle veggies evenly with garlic powder and season with salt and pepper. To assemble kebabs layer

steak and veggies onto kebabs in desired order; work to fit four steak pieces onto each kebab.

5. Brush grill grates lightly with oil. Place kebabs on grill and grill until center of steak registers about 140–145 degrees for medium doneness, turning kebabs occasionally, about eight to nine minutes. Serve warm.

## BAKED TURKEY QUINOA SPINACH MEATBALLS

*Ingredients*

2 lbs. lean ground turkey
1 cup cooked quinoa
1 medium yellow onion, diced very small
6 garlic cloves, minced
1 cup fresh chopped spinach leaves
2 tbsp. low sodium soy sauce, sriracha sauce,

or Worcestershire sauce
1 tbsp. dried Italian seasoning/spices
1 tsp. dried oregano
1 tbsp. ground flaxseed
Salt and pepper
1 egg, beaten

*Directions (Servings: 6)*

1. Preheat oven to 350°F and spray baking pan (with sides) with baking spray. Set aside.
2. In stand mixer with the paddle attached, add all ingredients and mix until incorporated.
3. Form meatballs, rolling between your hands and then lay out on baking sheet.
4. Repeat until all meat mixture is used.
5. Bake for thirty-five minutes or a little longer, until golden brown.

6. Rotate them halfway through the baking time.
7. Bake until fully cooked throughout.

## SPICY SALMON BOWL

### Salmon
*Ingredients*

1/4 cup low-sodium soy
   sauce
1/3 cup extra-virgin olive
   oil
4 tbsp. chili powder

Juice of 1 lime
2 tbsp. honey
4 cloves garlic, minced
4 salmon fillets (4 oz.
   each)

### Cucumbers
*Ingredients*

1/4 cup rice vinegar or
   rice wine vinegar
1 tsp. granulated sugar
1 tsp. kosher salt

2 tsp. toasted sesame oil
3 cucumbers, thinly
   sliced

### Spicy Mayo/Greek Yogurt
*Ingredients*

1/2 cup plain nonfat
   Greek yogurt

2 tbsp. Sriracha
2 tbsp. toasted sesame

### Bowls
*Ingredients*

3 cups cooked brown rice
1 avocado, sliced
1 medium carrot, grated

1/2 red onion,
   sliced
Cilantro leaves
Sesame seeds

steak and veggies onto kebabs in desired order; work to fit four steak pieces onto each kebab.

5. Brush grill grates lightly with oil. Place kebabs on grill and grill until center of steak registers about 140–145 degrees for medium doneness, turning kebabs occasionally, about eight to nine minutes. Serve warm.

## BAKED TURKEY QUINOA SPINACH MEATBALLS

*Ingredients*

2 lbs. lean ground turkey

1 cup cooked quinoa

1 medium yellow onion, diced very small

6 garlic cloves, minced

1 cup fresh chopped spinach leaves

2 tbsp. low sodium soy sauce, sriracha sauce, or Worcestershire sauce

1 tbsp. dried Italian seasoning/spices

1 tsp. dried oregano

1 tbsp. ground flaxseed

Salt and pepper

1 egg, beaten

*Directions (Servings: 6)*

1. Preheat oven to 350°F and spray baking pan (with sides) with baking spray. Set aside.

2. In stand mixer with the paddle attached, add all ingredients and mix until incorporated.

3. Form meatballs, rolling between your hands and then lay out on baking sheet.

4. Repeat until all meat mixture is used.

5. Bake for thirty-five minutes or a little longer, until golden brown.

6. Rotate them halfway through the baking time.
7. Bake until fully cooked throughout.

## SPICY SALMON BOWL

### Salmon
*Ingredients*

$1/3$ cup low-sodium soy sauce

$1/3$ cup extra virgin olive oil

3 tbsp. chili powder

Juice of 1 lime

2 tbsp. honey

4 cloves garlic, minced

4 salmon fillets (4 oz. each)

### Cucumbers
*Ingredients*

$1/2$ cup rice vinegar or rice wine vinegar

1 tsp. granulated sugar

1 tsp. kosher salt

2 tsp. toasted sesame oil

3 cucumbers, thinly sliced

### Spicy Mayo/Greek Yogurt
*Ingredients*

$1/2$ cup plain nonfat Greek yogurt

2 tbsp. sriracha

2 tbsp. toasted sesame oil

### Bowls
*Ingredients*

3 cups cooked brown rice

1 avocado, sliced

1 medium carrot, grated

$1/2$ red onion, thinly sliced

Cilantro leaves, torn

Sesame seeds

*Directions (Servings: 4)*

1. Preheat oven to 350° and line a large baking sheet with foil. In a medium bowl, whisk together soy sauce, olive oil, chili, lime juice, honey, and garlic. Add salmon and gently toss to combine. Place on prepared baking sheet and bake until salmon is fork-tender, twenty to twenty-five minutes.

2. In a microwave-safe bowl or jar, add vinegar, sugar, and salt and microwave until sugar and salt are dissolved, about two minutes. Stir in sesame oil, then add cucumbers and shake to combine. Cover with a tight-fitting lid or plastic wrap until ready to use.

3. In a small bowl, combine mayonnaise, sriracha, and sesame oil.

4. Divide rice among four bowls. Top with salmon, pickled cucumbers, avocado, carrot, red onion, cilantro, and sesame seeds. Drizzle with spicy mayo.

## MEDITERRANEAN PASTA SALAD

*Ingredients*

12 oz. dry pasta

1 English cucumber, diced

1 pint cherry or grape tomatoes, halved

2/3 cup sliced Kalamata olives

4 oz. crumbled feta cheese

1/2 of a medium red onion, peeled and thinly sliced

### Lemon-Herb Vinaigrette
*Ingredients*

1/4 cup extra virgin olive oil

3 tablespoons red wine vinegar

1 tbsp. freshly squeezed lemon juice

2 tsp. dried oregano, minced

1 tsp. honey (or your desired sweetener)

2 small garlic cloves, minced

1/4 tsp. freshly cracked black pepper

1/4 tsp. salt

Pinch of crushed red pepper flakes

*Directions (Servings: 6)*

1. Cook pasta al dente in a large stockpot according to package instructions. Drain pasta, then rinse under cold water for about twenty to thirty seconds until no longer hot. Transfer pasta to a large mixing bowl.

2. Add cucumber, tomatoes, Kalamata olives, feta cheese, and red onion to mixing bowl, then drizzle all of vinaigrette evenly on top. Toss until all ingredients are evenly coated with dressing.

3. Serve immediately, garnished with extra feta and black pepper if desired.

4. To make lemon-herb vinaigrette, whisk all ingredients together until combined.

## LOW-SODIUM TURKEY CHILI

*Ingredients*

1 lb. ground turkey, extra lean

3 garlic cloves, minced

2 medium onions, finely chopped

3 large celery stalks, chopped

2 medium bell peppers, chopped

14 oz. can low-sodium red kidney beans, drained and rinsed

14 oz. can low-sodium white beans, drained

and rinsed

28 oz. can tomato sauce or crushed tomatoes, low-sodium

1 cup chicken or vegetable broth, low-sodium

1 tbsp. red pepper flakes

1 tbsp. chili powder, low-sodium

1 tbsp. taco seasoning, low-sodium

Salt and ground black pepper to taste

Oil for frying

Lime, cilantro, cheese, yogurt, chips, etc. for serving

### Directions (Servings: 6)

1. Preheat large 5–6 quart Dutch oven, heavy bottom pot, or ceramic non-stick skillet on high heat, and add ground turkey. Cook until small pieces form, or about five minutes, stirring and breaking constantly into small pieces with spatula. Transfer to a bowl or large slow cooker and set aside.

2. Return skillet or pot to medium heat and swirl a bit of oil to coat. Add garlic and onion, sauté until translucent or five minutes, stirring occasionally. Add celery and bell peppers, sauté for five more minutes, stirring occasionally. If using slow cooker, transfer there, or leave in Dutch oven.

3. Then to either, add red kidney and white beans, tomato sauce, broth, chipotle pepper, chili powder, taco seasoning, and pepper.

4. Cover, bring to a boil, reduce heat to low, and simmer for about thirty minutes. In slow cooker, cook on low for eight hours or on high for four hours.

5. Stir and add salt to taste, if necessary. Serve warm with your favorite toppings!

# Dietary Analysis

| WEEK ONE | | | | |
|---|---|---|---|---|
| **BREAKFAST** | **LUNCH** | **SNACK** | **DINNER** | **TOTALS** |
| **MONDAY**<br>Calories: 430<br>Carbs: 50g<br>Protein: 36g<br>Fat: 11g<br>Fiber: 12g<br>Sodium: 430mg | Calories: 300<br>Carbs: 46g<br>Protein: 14g<br>Fat: 8g<br>Fiber: 8g<br>Sodium: 502mg | Calories: 116<br>Carbs: 13g<br>Protein: 4g<br>Fat: 5g<br>Fiber: 4g<br>Sodium: 131mg | Calories: 286<br>Carbs: 14g<br>Protein: 19g<br>Fat: 10g<br>Fiber: 4g<br>Sodium: 293mg | Calories: 1,132<br>Carbs: 123g<br>Protein: 73g<br>Fat: 34g<br>Fiber: 28g<br>Sodium: 1,356mg |
| **TUESDAY**<br>Calories: 451<br>Carbs: 56g<br>Protein: 18g<br>Fat: 20g<br>Fiber: 14g<br>Sodium: 416mg | Calories: 292<br>Carbs: 10g<br>Protein: 9g<br>Fat: 20g<br>Fiber: 7g<br>Sodium: 69mg | Calories: 315<br>Carbs: 43g<br>Protein: 8g<br>Fat: 15g<br>Fiber: 4g<br>Sodium: 115mg | Calories: 426<br>Carbs: 25g<br>Protein: 20g<br>Fat: 21g<br>Fiber: 4g<br>Sodium: 570mg | Calories: 1,484<br>Carbs: 134g<br>Protein: 55g<br>Fat: 76g<br>Fiber: 29g<br>Sodium: 1,170mg |
| **WEDNESDAY**<br>Calories: 339<br>Carbs: 28g<br>Protein: 29g<br>Fat: 14g<br>Fiber: 7g<br>Sodium: 107mg | Calories: 354<br>Carbs: 38g<br>Protein: 10g<br>Fat: 18g<br>Fiber: 4g<br>Sodium: 322mg | Calories: 202<br>Carbs: 16g<br>Protein: 7g<br>Fat: 14g<br>Fiber: 6g<br>Sodium: 1mg | Calories: 612<br>Carbs: 63g<br>Protein: 37g<br>Fat: 27g<br>Fiber: 12g<br>Sodium: 611mg | Calories: 1,507<br>Carbs: 145g<br>Protein: 83g<br>Fat: 73g<br>Fiber: 29g<br>Sodium: 1,041mg |
| **THURSDAY**<br>Calories: 412<br>Carbs: 46g<br>Protein: 11g<br>Fat: 22g<br>Fiber: 11g<br>Sodium: 79mg | Calories: 367<br>Carbs: 40g<br>Protein: 26g<br>Fat: 12g<br>Fiber: 6g<br>Sodium: 540mg | Calories: 346<br>Carbs: 56g<br>Protein: 8g<br>Fat: 13g<br>Fiber: 7g<br>Sodium: 208mg | Calories: 490<br>Carbs: 22g<br>Protein: 29g<br>Fat: 33g<br>Fiber: 5g<br>Sodium: 487mg | Calories: 1,615<br>Carbs: 164g<br>Protein: 164g<br>Fat: 80g<br>Fiber: 29g<br>Sodium: 1,314mg |
| **FRIDAY**<br>Calories: 440<br>Carbs: 14g<br>Protein: 31g<br>Fat: 29g<br>Fiber: 6g<br>Sodium: 393mg | Calories: 524<br>Carbs: 75g<br>Protein: 19g<br>Fat: 20g<br>Fiber: 16g<br>Sodium: 517mg | Calories: 93<br>Carbs: 18g<br>Protein: 3g<br>Fat: 1g<br>Fiber: 4g<br>Sodium: 2mg | Calories: 250<br>Carbs: 30g<br>Protein: 11g<br>Fat: 4g<br>Fiber: 11g<br>Sodium: 302mg | Calories: 1,307<br>Carbs: 137g<br>Protein: 64g<br>Fat: 54g<br>Fiber: 37g<br>Sodium: 1,214mg |
| **SATURDAY**<br>Calories: 390<br>Carbs: 47g<br>Protein: 32g<br>Fat: 11g<br>Fiber: 13g<br>Sodium: 361mg | Calories: 371<br>Carbs: 44g<br>Protein: 29g<br>Fat: 8g<br>Fiber: 10g<br>Sodium: 759mg | Calories: 331<br>Carbs: 44g<br>Protein: 8g<br>Fat: 16g<br>Fiber: 9g<br>Sodium: 158mg | Calories: 555<br>Carbs: 48g<br>Protein: 25g<br>Fat: 29g<br>Fiber: 3g<br>Sodium: 635mg | Calories: 1,647<br>Carbs: 183g<br>Protein: 94g<br>Fat: 64g<br>Fiber: 35g<br>Sodium: 1,913mg |
| **SUNDAY**<br>Calories: 395<br>Carbs: 33g<br>Protein: 17g<br>Fat: 23g<br>Fiber: 5g<br>Sodium: 1mg | Calories: 364<br>Carbs: 33g<br>Protein: 29g<br>Fat: 10g<br>Fiber: 6g<br>Sodium: 681mg | Calories: 349<br>Carbs: 54g<br>Protein: 8g<br>Fat: 14g<br>Fiber: 8g<br>Sodium: 18mg | Calories: 290<br>Carbs: 39g<br>Protein: 16g<br>Fat: 8g<br>Fiber: 6g<br>Sodium: 632mg | Calories: 1,398<br>Carbs: 159g<br>Protein: 70g<br>Fat: 55g<br>Fiber: 25g<br>Sodium: 1,332mg |

| WEEK TWO | | | | |
|---|---|---|---|---|
| | BREAKFAST | LUNCH | SNACK | DINNER | TOTALS |

| | BREAKFAST | LUNCH | SNACK | DINNER | TOTALS |
|---|---|---|---|---|---|
| **MONDAY** | Calories: 494<br>Carbs: 88g<br>Protein: 19g<br>Fat: 9g<br>Fiber: 12g<br>Sodium: 126mg | Calories: 498<br>Carbs: 46g<br>Protein: 21g<br>Fat: 27g<br>Fiber: 12g<br>Sodium: 360mg | Calories: 116<br>Carbs: 20g<br>Protein: 4g<br>Fat: 3g<br>Fiber: 9g<br>Sodium: 262mg | Calories: 440<br>Carbs: 15g<br>Protein: 32g<br>Fat: 27g<br>Fiber: 4g<br>Sodium: 700mg | Calories: 1,548<br>Carbs: 169g<br>Protein: 76g<br>Fat: 66g<br>Fiber: 37g<br>Sodium: 1,448mg |
| **TUESDAY** | Calories: 518<br>Carbs: 72g<br>Protein: 19g<br>Fat: 17g<br>Fiber: 14g<br>Sodium: 355mg | Calories: 444<br>Carbs: 54g<br>Protein: 12g<br>Fat: 22g<br>Fiber: 10g<br>Sodium: 611mg | Calories: 225<br>Carbs: 22g<br>Protein: 8g<br>Fat: 14g<br>Fiber: 7g<br>Sodium: 1mg | Calories: 438<br>Carbs: 37g<br>Protein: 54g<br>Fat: 8g<br>Fiber: 9g<br>Sodium: 272mg | Calories: 1,625<br>Carbs: 185g<br>Protein: 93g<br>Fat: 61g<br>Fiber: 40g<br>Sodium: 1,239mg |
| **WEDNESDAY** | Calories: 578<br>Carbs: 65g<br>Protein: 36g<br>Fat: 22g<br>Fiber: 10g<br>Sodium: 542mg | Calories: 422<br>Carbs: 46g<br>Protein: 22g<br>Fat: 17g<br>Fiber: 12g<br>Sodium: 603mg | Calories: 175<br>Carbs: 25g<br>Protein: 6g<br>Fat: 7g<br>Fiber: 5g<br>Sodium: 142mg | Calories: 390<br>Carbs: 16g<br>Protein: 41g<br>Fat: 18g<br>Fiber: 5g<br>Sodium: 272mg | Calories: 1,565<br>Carbs: 152g<br>Protein: 105g<br>Fat: 64g<br>Fiber: 32g<br>Sodium: 1,559mg |
| **THURSDAY** | Calories: 310<br>Carbs: 41g<br>Protein: 8g<br>Fat: 15g<br>Fiber: 10g<br>Sodium: 171mg | Calories: 515<br>Carbs: 49g<br>Protein: 20g<br>Fat: 26g<br>Fiber: 14g<br>Sodium: 564mg | Calories: 278<br>Carbs: 19g<br>Protein: 25g<br>Fat: 12g<br>Fiber: 4g<br>Sodium: 580mg | Calories: 343<br>Carbs: 29g<br>Protein: 26g<br>Fat: 13g<br>Fiber: 5g<br>Sodium: 520mg | Calories: 1,446<br>Carbs: 138g<br>Protein: 79g<br>Fat: 66g<br>Fiber: 33g<br>Sodium: 1,835mg |
| **FRIDAY** | Calories: 585<br>Carbs: 57g<br>Protein: 33g<br>Fat: 24g<br>Fiber: 15g<br>Sodium: 608mg | Calories: 399<br>Carbs: 42g<br>Protein: 40g<br>Fat: 5g<br>Fiber: 6g<br>Sodium: 182mg | Calories: 231<br>Carbs: 15g<br>Protein: 6g<br>Fat: 18g<br>Fiber: 6g<br>Sodium: 2mg | Calories: 528<br>Carbs: 45g<br>Protein: 21g<br>Fat: 17g<br>Fiber: 9g<br>Sodium: 485mg | Calories: 1,743<br>Carbs: 159g<br>Protein: 100g<br>Fat: 64g<br>Fiber: 36g<br>Sodium: 1,277mg |
| **SATURDAY** | Calories: 491<br>Carbs: 60g<br>Protein: 15g<br>Fat: 23g<br>Fiber: 11g<br>Sodium: 160mg | Calories: 440<br>Carbs: 30g<br>Protein: 34g<br>Fat: 21g<br>Fiber: 6g<br>Sodium: 546mg | Calories: 431<br>Carbs: 39g<br>Protein: 14g<br>Fat: 28g<br>Fiber: 12g<br>Sodium: 299mg | Calories: 535<br>Carbs: 23g<br>Protein: 12g<br>Fat: 24g<br>Fiber: 5g<br>Sodium: 408mg | Calories: 1,897<br>Carbs: 152g<br>Protein: 75g<br>Fat: 96g<br>Fiber: 34g<br>Sodium: 1,413mg |
| **SUNDAY** | Calories: 397<br>Carbs: 65g<br>Protein: 20g<br>Fat: 6g<br>Fiber: 15g<br>Sodium: 420mg | Calories: 483<br>Carbs: 48g<br>Protein: 11g<br>Fat: 18g<br>Fiber: 12g<br>Sodium: 320mg | Calories: 207<br>Carbs: 29g<br>Protein: 8g<br>Fat: 6g<br>Fiber: 9g<br>Sodium: 415mg | Calories: 205<br>Carbs: 4g<br>Protein: 27g<br>Fat: 9g<br>Fiber: 1g<br>Sodium: 271mg | Calories: 1,292<br>Carbs: 146g<br>Protein: 66g<br>Fat: 39g<br>Fiber: 37g<br>Sodium: 1,426mg |

| | | | WEEK THREE | | |
|---|---|---|---|---|---|
| | BREAKFAST | LUNCH | SNACK | DINNER | TOTALS |
| **MONDAY** | Calories: 399<br>Carbs: 65g<br>Protein: 15g<br>Fat: 11g<br>Fiber: 12g<br>Sodium: 248mg | Calories: 310<br>Carbs: 30g<br>Protein: 20g<br>Fat: 17g<br>Fiber: 13g<br>Sodium: 623mg | Calories: 394<br>Carbs: 24g<br>Protein: 14g<br>Fat: 28g<br>Fiber: 10g<br>Sodium: 78mg | Calories: 430<br>Carbs: 15g<br>Protein: 50g<br>Fat: 19g<br>Fiber: 5g<br>Sodium: 532mg | Calories: 1,533<br>Carbs: 134g<br>Protein: 99g<br>Fat: 75g<br>Fiber: 40g<br>Sodium: 1,481mg |
| **TUESDAY** | Calories: 537<br>Carbs: 50g<br>Protein: 25g<br>Fat: 20g<br>Fiber: 14g<br>Sodium: 423mg | Calories: 473<br>Carbs: 53g<br>Protein: 13g<br>Fat: 26g<br>Fiber: 8g<br>Sodium: 361mg | Calories: 132<br>Carbs: 15g<br>Protein: 6g<br>Fat: 5g<br>Fiber: 4g<br>Sodium: 85mg | Calories: 348<br>Carbs: 32g<br>Protein: 27g<br>Fat: 14g<br>Fiber: 7g<br>Sodium: 493mg | Calories: 1,490<br>Carbs: 150g<br>Protein: 71g<br>Fat: 65g<br>Fiber: 33g<br>Sodium: 1,362mg |
| **WEDNESDAY** | Calories: 384<br>Carbs: 37g<br>Protein: 30g<br>Fat: 14g<br>Fiber: 8g<br>Sodium: 207mg | Calories: 650<br>Carbs: 84g<br>Protein: 18g<br>Fat: 28g<br>Fiber: 20g<br>Sodium: 337mg | Calories: 239<br>Carbs: 22g<br>Protein: 7g<br>Fat: 15g<br>Fiber: 6g<br>Sodium: 317mg | Calories: 533<br>Carbs: 36g<br>Protein: 29g<br>Fat: 31g<br>Fiber: 11g<br>Sodium: 465mg | Calories: 1,806<br>Carbs: 179g<br>Protein: 84g<br>Fat: 88g<br>Fiber: 45g<br>Sodium: 1,326mg |
| **THURSDAY** | Calories: 324<br>Carbs: 24g<br>Protein: 23g<br>Fat: 16g<br>Fiber: 8g<br>Sodium: 620mg | Calories: 757<br>Carbs: 72g<br>Protein: 63g<br>Fat: 21g<br>Fiber: 6g<br>Sodium: 623mg | Calories: 238<br>Carbs: 29g<br>Protein: 8g<br>Fat: 9g<br>Fiber: 8g<br>Sodium: 326mg | Calories: 497<br>Carbs: 42g<br>Protein: 10g<br>Fat: 23g<br>Fiber: 8g<br>Sodium: 270mg | Calories: 1,816<br>Carbs: 167g<br>Protein: 104g<br>Fat: 69g<br>Fiber: 30g<br>Sodium: 1,839mg |
| **FRIDAY** | Calories: 565<br>Carbs: 74g<br>Protein: 15g<br>Fat: 25g<br>Fiber: 15g<br>Sodium: 321mg | Calories: 497<br>Carbs: 42g<br>Protein: 10g<br>Fat: 23g<br>Fiber: 8g<br>Sodium: 470mg | Calories: 193<br>Carbs: 30g<br>Protein: 3g<br>Fat: 5g<br>Fiber: 5g<br>Sodium: 121mg | Calories: 389<br>Carbs: 32g<br>Protein: 30g<br>Fat: 16g<br>Fiber: 5g<br>Sodium: 489mg | Calories: 1,644<br>Carbs: 178g<br>Protein: 58g<br>Fat: 69g<br>Fiber: 33g<br>Sodium: 1,401mg |
| **SATURDAY** | Calories: 450<br>Carbs: 36g<br>Protein: 17g<br>Fat: 17g<br>Fiber: 5g<br>Sodium: 349mg | Calories: 620<br>Carbs: 56g<br>Protein: 22g<br>Fat: 37g<br>Fiber: 19g<br>Sodium: 639mg | Calories: 251<br>Carbs: 59g<br>Protein: 8g<br>Fat: 1g<br>Fiber: 7g<br>Sodium: 132mg | Calories: 263<br>Carbs: 29g<br>Protein: 24g<br>Fat: 6g<br>Fiber: 6g<br>Sodium: 366mg | Calories: 1,584<br>Carbs: 180g<br>Protein: 71g<br>Fat: 61g<br>Fiber: 37g<br>Sodium: 1,486mg |
| **SUNDAY** | Calories: 366<br>Carbs: 41g<br>Protein: 14g<br>Fat: 18g<br>Fiber: 11g<br>Sodium: 291mg | Calories: 534<br>Carbs: 9g<br>Protein: 41g<br>Fat: 36g<br>Fiber: 5g<br>Sodium: 519mg | Calories: 181<br>Carbs: 23g<br>Protein: 5g<br>Fat: 9g<br>Fiber: 4g<br>Sodium: 138mg | Calories: 356<br>Carbs: 46g<br>Protein: 13g<br>Fat: 15g<br>Fiber: 9g<br>Sodium: 531mg | Calories: 1,437<br>Carbs: 119g<br>Protein: 73g<br>Fat: 78g<br>Fiber: 29g<br>Sodium: 1479mg |

| WEEK FOUR | | | | |
|---|---|---|---|---|
| | BREAKFAST | LUNCH | SNACK | DINNER | TOTALS |

| | BREAKFAST | LUNCH | SNACK | DINNER | TOTALS |
|---|---|---|---|---|---|
| **MONDAY** | Calories: 398<br>Carbs: 48g<br>Protein: 23g<br>Fat: 13g<br>Fiber: 12g<br>Sodium: 397mg | Calories: 629<br>Carbs: 49g<br>Protein: 40g<br>Fat: 33g<br>Fiber: 11g<br>Sodium: 456mg | Calories: 336<br>Carbs: 35g<br>Protein: 22g<br>Fat: 12g<br>Fiber: 7g<br>Sodium: 540mg | Calories: 182<br>Carbs: 10g<br>Protein: 18g<br>Fat: 8g<br>Fiber: 2g<br>Sodium: 621mg | Calories: 1,545<br>Carbs: 142g<br>Protein: 103g<br>Fat: 66g<br>Fiber: 32g<br>Sodium: 2,014mg |
| **TUESDAY** | Calories: 466<br>Carbs: 43g<br>Protein: 34g<br>Fat: 19g<br>Fiber: 7g<br>Sodium: 456mg | Calories: 413<br>Carbs: 15g<br>Protein: 55g<br>Fat: 15g<br>Fiber: 4g<br>Sodium: 632mg | Calories: 454<br>Carbs: 75g<br>Protein: 2g<br>Fat: 7g<br>Fiber: 9g<br>Sodium: 206mg | Calories: 320<br>Carbs: 22g<br>Protein: 13g<br>Fat: 20g<br>Fiber: 6g<br>Sodium: 340mg | Calories: 1,653<br>Carbs: 155g<br>Protein: 104g<br>Fat: 61g<br>Fiber: 24g<br>Sodium: 1,634mg |
| **WEDNESDAY** | Calories: 510<br>Carbs: 49g<br>Protein: 37g<br>Fat: 17g<br>Fiber: 9g<br>Sodium: 200mg | Calories: 301<br>Carbs: 23g<br>Protein: 22g<br>Fat: 14g<br>Fiber: 6g<br>Sodium: 363mg | Calories: 456<br>Carbs: 65g<br>Protein: 11g<br>Fat: 19g<br>Fiber: 13g<br>Sodium: 153mg | Calories: 353<br>Carbs: 18g<br>Protein: 34g<br>Fat: 14g<br>Fiber: 3g<br>Sodium: 588mg | Calories: 1,620<br>Carbs: 155g<br>Protein: 104g<br>Fat: 64g<br>Fiber: 31g<br>Sodium: 1,304mg |
| **THURSDAY** | Calories: 416<br>Carbs: 62g<br>Protein: 29g<br>Fat: 7g<br>Fiber: 11g<br>Sodium: 351mg | Calories: 550<br>Carbs: 18g<br>Protein: 32g<br>Fat: 29g<br>Fiber: 5g<br>Sodium: 435mg | Calories: 387<br>Carbs: 45g<br>Protein: 17g<br>Fat: 18g<br>Fiber: 4g<br>Sodium: 240mg | Calories: 269<br>Carbs: 35g<br>Protein: 23g<br>Fat: 3g<br>Fiber: 3g<br>Sodium: 239mg | Calories: 1,622<br>Carbs: 160g<br>Protein: 101g<br>Fat: 57g<br>Fiber: 23g<br>Sodium: 1,265mg |
| **FRIDAY** | Calories: 294<br>Carbs: 6g<br>Protein: 24g<br>Fat: 4g<br>Fiber: 2g<br>Sodium: 230mg | Calories: 351<br>Carbs: 18g<br>Protein: 22g<br>Fat: 16g<br>Fiber: 8g<br>Sodium: 148mg | Calories: 253<br>Carbs: 23g<br>Protein: 28g<br>Fat: 6g<br>Fiber: 3g<br>Sodium: 451mg | Calories: 430<br>Carbs: 46g<br>Protein: 31g<br>Fat: 13g<br>Fiber: 4g<br>Sodium: 650mg | Calories: 1,328<br>Carbs: 93g<br>Protein: 105g<br>Fat: 39g<br>Fiber: 17g<br>Sodium: 1,479mg |
| **SATURDAY** | Calories: 512<br>Carbs: 53g<br>Protein: 33g<br>Fat: 21g<br>Fiber: 14g<br>Sodium: 563mg | Calories: 425<br>Carbs: 48g<br>Protein: 17g<br>Fat: 18g<br>Fiber: 11g<br>Sodium: 295mg | Calories: 284<br>Carbs: 47g<br>Protein: 25g<br>Fat: 1g<br>Fiber: 6g<br>Sodium: 110mg | Calories: 378<br>Carbs: 38g<br>Protein: 11g<br>Fat: 20g<br>Fiber: 6g<br>Sodium: 772mg | Calories: 1,599<br>Carbs: 186g<br>Protein: 86g<br>Fat: 60g<br>Fiber: 37g<br>Sodium: 1,740mg |
| **SUNDAY** | Calories: 661<br>Carbs: 83g<br>Protein: 24g<br>Fat: 30g<br>Fiber: 14g<br>Sodium: 115mg | Calories: 448<br>Carbs: 28g<br>Protein: 8g<br>Fat: 35g<br>Fiber: 6g<br>Sodium: 782mg | Calories: 275<br>Carbs: 23g<br>Protein: 10g<br>Fat: 17g<br>Fiber: 11g<br>Sodium: 216mg | Calories: 347<br>Carbs: 42g<br>Protein: 34g<br>Fat: 5g<br>Fiber: 10g<br>Sodium: 129mg | Calories: 1,731<br>Carbs: 176g<br>Protein: 76g<br>Fat: 87g<br>Fiber: 41g<br>Sodium: 1,242mg |

---

# Sample Grocery List

## *WEEK ONE*

### PRODUCE

- ❏ 10 oz. container baby spinach
- ❏ 16 oz. container strawberries
- ❏ 6 oz. container raspberries
- ❏ 2 pints blueberries
- ❏ 6 oz. container blackberries
- ❏ 1 large tomato
- ❏ 2 plum tomatoes
- ❏ 4 red onions
- ❏ 1 red pepper
- ❏ 1 yellow onion
- ❏ 1 cucumber
- ❏ 1 avocado
- ❏ 5 oz. container or bag of arugula
- ❏ 5 oz. container or bag of kale
- ❏ 1 red cabbage
- ❏ 1 lb. bag carrots
- ❏ 1 banana
- ❏ 1 small head of romaine
- ❏ 2 bell peppers
- ❏ 2 mangos
- ❏ 1 pineapple
- ❏ 2 kiwis
- ❏ 2 cups fresh cherries
- ❏ 1 large apple
- ❏ 3 lemons
- ❏ 1 lb. green beans
- ❏ 1 orange
- ❏ 1 garlic bulb
- ❏ 1 small ginger
- ❏ 1 green onion head
- ❏ 2 lbs. butternut squash
- ❏ 2 containers baby portabella mushrooms (8 oz. each)
- ❏ 1 shallot
- ❏ 1 medium zucchini
- ❏ Fresh sage, 8 leaves
- ❏ 1/4 cup sundried tomatoes (from salad bar)

## PANTRY

- ❏ 16 oz. bottle extra virgin olive oil
- ❏ Small bag ground flaxseed
- ❏ Choice of salad dressing or Italian
- ❏ Low-fat mayo
- ❏ 1 jar natural jam, choice of flavor
- ❏ 1 small bag trail mix, low-sugar
- ❏ 1 small bottle dry white wine, 5–6 oz.
- ❏ 1 small bottle balsamic vinegar
- ❏ 1 container orange juice
- ❏ 1 small bag brown sugar
- ❏ Low-sodium soy sauce
- ❏ Sesame oil
- ❏ Sesame seeds
- ❏ 1 can, diced green chiles
- ❏ 1 jar pesto
- ❏ 1 can black beans with no salt added

## WHOLE GRAINS

- ❏ 1 loaf whole-grain bread
- ❏ 1 container dried oats
- ❏ 1 bag tortilla wraps
- ❏ 1 box whole-grain crackers
- ❏ 1 large bag air-popped popcorn
- ❏ 5 whole pita breads
- ❏ 1 loaf ciabatta bread (14 oz.)

## PROTEIN

- ❏ 1 dozen eggs
- ❏ 1 jar choice of nut butter
- ❏ 3 oz. chopped walnuts
- ❏ 10 oz. container red pepper hummus
- ❏ 1 packet tuna in water, low-sodium
- ❏ 1 package low-sodium turkey breast
- ❏ 3 oz. almonds
- ❏ 1 oz. pistachios

❑ 4 portion salmon fillets (6 oz. each)

❑ 1 ¹/₂ lbs. top sirloin steak
❑ 1 ¹/₂ lbs. sea scallops

## DAIRY

❑ 1 small bag low-fat shredded cheese, any flavor
❑ 32 oz. plain low-fat Greek yogurt
❑ ¹/₂ gallon unsweetened almond milk
❑ 1 small bag cheddar cheese
❑ 1 pint low-fat milk
❑ ¹/₄ pound sliced low-fat cheese, any flavor

❑ 1 small container low-fat cottage cheese
❑ 1 small container half-and-half
❑ 1 small container unsalted butter
❑ 2 cups shredded mozzarella cheese
❑ 1 small bag low-fat Monterey jack cheese, shredded
❑ 1 package crumbled feta cheese

## MISCELLANEOUS

❑ Cinnamon
❑ Pure vanilla extract
❑ Salt
❑ Pepper

❑ Garlic powder
❑ Skewers
❑ Cayenne pepper

## WEEK TWO

## PRODUCE

❑ 2 pints blueberries
❑ 1 nectarine
❑ 7 bell peppers, any color
❑ 2 onions

❑ 1 red onion
❑ 1 shallot
❑ 1 container mushrooms
❑ 1 apple or pear

- ❏ 5 bananas
- ❏ 10 oz. bag salad mix
- ❏ 5 oz. baby arugula
- ❏ 10 oz. bag/container spring mix
- ❏ 5 oz. bag/container kale
- ❏ ½ lb. string beans
- ❏ 5 heads broccoli
- ❏ 1 small head cabbage
- ❏ 10 oz. container baby spinach
- ❏ 1 cup melon, or choice of fruit
- ❏ 3 cups shredded romaine lettuce
- ❏ 3 medium-large tomatoes
- ❏ 1 cucumber
- ❏ 1 kiwi
- ❏ 3 apples
- ❏ 6 oz. container raspberries
- ❏ 2 lb. bag carrots
- ❏ 2 avocados
- ❏ 2 bags baby carrots
- ❏ 1 orange
- ❏ 2 containers of strawberries (16 oz. each)
- ❏ 3 lemons
- ❏ 1 sweet potato
- ❏ 2 garlic bulbs
- ❏ 12 oz. grape tomatoes
- ❏ 3 scallions
- ❏ 6 oz. marinated artichoke hearts

## PANTRY

- ❏ Salad dressing, your choice
- ❏ Flaxseed or olive oil, 16 oz. bottle
- ❏ Choice of vinegar
- ❏ 1 can low-sodium chickpeas
- ❏ 1 container panko bread crumbs
- ❏ 1 jar pesto
- ❏ 1 small bag shredded unsweetened coconut
- ❏ 1 box corn starch
- ❏ 1 box low-sodium chicken broth
- ❏ Low-sodium soy sauce
- ❏ 1 jar honey
- ❏ Sesame oil
- ❏ BBQ sauce
- ❏ Ketchup
- ❏ Canola oil
- ❏ Brown sugar
- ❏ 1 jar pitted olives

## WHOLE GRAINS

- ❏ 1 container dried oats
- ❏ 1 box whole-grain cereal
- ❏ 1 box whole-grain waffles
- ❏ 1 loaf whole-grain bread
- ❏ 1 small bag pita bread
- ❏ 1 small bag brown rice
- ❏ 1 bag quinoa
- ❏ 1 bag farro
- ❏ 1 small bag ground flaxseed
- ❏ 1 small bag chia seeds
- ❏ 1 small container low-sugar granola
- ❏ Whole-grain hamburger buns
- ❏ 1 box whole-grain spaghetti

## PROTEIN

- ❏ 4 oz. almonds
- ❏ 1 jar nut butter
- ❏ 1 dozen eggs
- ❏ 1 salmon pouch
- ❏ 1 small bag sunflower seeds, shells removed
- ❏ 10 oz. container hummus
- ❏ 2 oz. mixed nuts
- ❏ 2 oz. walnuts
- ❏ 6 oz. fresh salmon
- ❏ 1 1/2 lbs. of cod or haddock
- ❏ 1 1/2 lbs. boneless, skinless chicken breasts
- ❏ 1 1/4 lbs. lean ground turkey
- ❏ 1 1/4 lbs. skinless halibut fillets

## DAIRY

- ❏ 1/2 gallon low-fat milk
- ❏ 1/2 gallon unsweetened vanilla almond milk
- ❏ 6 oz. vanilla low-fat Greek yogurt
- ❏ 8 oz. plain low-fat Greek yogurt
- ❏ 1 small bag low-fat shredded cheese
- ❏ 1 package crumbled feta cheese
- ❏ 2 cups cottage cheese
- ❏ 1 bag cheese sticks
- ❏ 4 oz. goat cheese

## FROZEN

❏ 1 cup shelled edamame ❏ 1 cup mixed berries

## MISCELLANEOUS

❏ Fresh or dried thyme ❏ Fresh ginger
❏ Fresh or dried rosemary ❏ Tarragon
❏ Red pepper flakes ❏ Salt
❏ 1 1/2 cups fresh parsley ❏ Pepper
❏ 10–15 fresh basil leaves ❏ Coconut flakes

### *WEEK THREE*

## PRODUCE

❏ 1 pear ❏ 1 pineapple
❏ 2 oranges ❏ 1 mango
❏ 10 tomatoes ❏ 7 lemons
❏ 10 oz. container ❏ 3 white or yellow onions
baby spinach ❏ 1 small bag
❏ 5 avocados shredded lettuce
❏ 1 pint blueberries ❏ 4 small–medium
❏ 2 containers zucchini
strawberries (16 ❏ 3 small–medium
oz. each) yellow squash
❏ 2 cucumbers ❏ 2 garlic bulbs
❏ 5 oz. container ❏ 1 medium spaghetti
spring mix greens squash
❏ 1 lb. bag carrots ❏ 1/2 lb. sliced mushrooms
❏ 5 red onions ❏ 1 cucumber
❏ Fresh basil leaves ❏ 4 heads broccoli
❏ 1 head romaine lettuce ❏ 1 1/2 cup grape tomatoes
❏ 9 bell peppers, any color ❏ 1 shallot
❏ 1 banana

## PANTRY

- ❏ 1 can beets
- ❏ 1 cup dried cherries
- ❏ Raspberry vinaigrette
- ❏ Red wine vinegar
- ❏ Mayo
- ❏ 16 oz. bottle olive oil
- ❏ Small bottle flaxseed oil
- ❏ Kale chips, any flavor
- ❏ Mini chocolate chips
- ❏ Unsweetened shredded coconut, small bag
- ❏ 1 can diced tomatoes, low-sodium, 14 oz.
- ❏ 1 jar pesto
- ❏ 1 container dry breadcrumbs
- ❏ 1 box low-sodium chicken broth
- ❏ Red wine vinegar
- ❏ 1 jar black olives
- ❏ 1 jar honey
- ❏ Low-sodium soy sauce
- ❏ Balsamic vinegar
- ❏ 1 small bag roasted edamame

## WHOLE GRAINS

- ❏ 1 loaf whole-grain bread
- ❏ 1 container plain oats
- ❏ Whole-grain English muffins
- ❏ Whole wheat pita bread
- ❏ 6" baguette
- ❏ 1 box whole-grain crackers
- ❏ Corn tortilla wraps
- ❏ Sourdough bread loaf
- ❏ 1 box dry penne pasta (16 oz.)

## PROTEIN

- ❏ Unsalted sliced almonds, small bag
- ❏ ½ dozen eggs
- ❏ 5 oz. almonds
- ❏ 2 jars nut butter
- ❏ 10 oz. container hummus
- ❏ 1 small bag sunflower seeds, shells removed
- ❏ 1 tuna pouch in oil

- ❏ 2 ¹/₂ lbs. boneless, skinless chicken breast
- ❏ 1–2 oz. mixed nuts
- ❏ 6 oz. fresh cod
- ❏ 2 lbs. peeled, deveined raw shrimp
- ❏ 1 package of smoked salmon
- ❏ 4 salmon fillets (6 oz. each)

## DAIRY

- ❏ 1 small container low-fat ricotta cheese
- ❏ 1 package crumbled feta cheese
- ❏ 6 oz. plain Greek low-fat yogurt
- ❏ 1 pint low-fat milk
- ❏ 1 small container goat cheese
- ❏ ¹/₄ lb. sliced provolone cheese
- ❏ 1 small container/ package fresh mozzarella
- ❏ 1 small bag low-fat shredded cheese, any flavor
- ❏ 1 small container butter
- ❏ 1 bag shredded parmesan cheese

## MISCELLANEOUS

- ❏ Paprika
- ❏ Cajun seasoning
- ❏ Fresh parsley
- ❏ Garlic powder
- ❏ Italian seasoning
- ❏ Dried or fresh oregano
- ❏ Dried or fresh dill
- ❏ Red pepper flakes
- ❏ Salt
- ❏ Pepper
- ❏ Dijon mustard

## *WEEK FOUR*

### PRODUCE

- ❏ 3 bananas
- ❏ 10 oz. container spinach
- ❏ 16 oz. container strawberries
- ❏ 3 tomatoes
- ❏ 4 apples
- ❏ 3 lemons
- ❏ 1 head celery
- ❏ 1 orange
- ❏ ½ cup shredded lettuce
- ❏ 10 oz. mixed greens
- ❏ 2 red cabbages
- ❏ 1 cucumber
- ❏ 2 lb. bag carrots
- ❏ 1 small bag kale
- ❏ 1 head cauliflower
- ❏ 7 bell peppers, any color
- ❏ 6 oz. container blueberries
- ❏ 2 mangos
- ❏ 6 oz. container blackberries or raspberries
- ❏ 3 garlic bulbs
- ❏ 1 jalapeño
- ❏ 5 white or yellow onions
- ❏ 2 heads broccoli
- ❏ 1 zucchini
- ❏ 8 oz. button mushrooms
- ❏ 3 red onions
- ❏ 2 limes
- ❏ 4 cucumbers or English cucumbers
- ❏ 1 avocado
- ❏ 2 cups grape tomatoes

### PANTRY

- ❏ 1 small bag ground flaxseed
- ❏ 1 small container/box low-sugar granola
- ❏ Mayo
- ❏ 1 small bag dried cranberries
- ❏ Low-sodium ginger and soy dressing
- ❏ Low-sodium soy sauce
- ❏ Rice vinegar
- ❏ 10 oz. 100% fruit juice or orange juice
- ❏ 1 small bag dried blueberries

❑ 1 small bag dried cherries

❑ 1 small bag trail mix, low-sugar

❑ 16 oz. bottle olive oil

❑ Red wine vinegar

❑ 1 small container Worcestershire sauce

❑ 1 jar honey

❑ 14 oz. can low-sodium red kidney beans

❑ 14 oz. can low-sodium white beans

❑ 28 oz. can tomato sauce, low-sodium

❑ 1 box chicken or vegetable broth, low-sodium

❑ Sesame oil

❑ 1 jar Kalamata olives

## WHOLE GRAINS

❑ 1 loaf whole-grain bread

❑ 1 small baguette loaf

❑ Whole-grain English muffins

❑ 1 container dry oats

❑ Whole-grain pita bread

❑ 2 cups dried whole-grain rice

❑ 1 box whole-grain crackers

❑ 8 small flour or corn tortilla shells

❑ 1 package dried quinoa

❑ 1 small bag ground flaxseed

❑ 1 bag whole-grain tortilla chips

❑ 16 oz. box dry pasta

## PROTEIN

❑ 1 dozen eggs

❑ 1 oz. chopped almonds

❑ Protein powder, your choice

❑ 1/2 lb. low-sodium turkey

❑ 3 oz. chopped walnuts

❑ 1 can low-sodium salmon

❑ 1 1/2 lbs. boneless, skinless chicken breast

- ❏ 1 oz. pecans
- ❏ 10 oz. container hummus
- ❏ 1 oz. pistachios
- ❏ 1 jar nut butter
- ❏ 1 oz. almonds
- ❏ 1 lb. raw shrimp
- ❏ 2 lbs. sirloin steak
- ❏ 3 lbs. lean ground turkey
- ❏ 4 salmon fillets (4 oz. each)
- ❏ 1 oz. sesame seeds

## DAIRY

- ❏ ½ gallon almond or cow's milk
- ❏ 1 large container low-fat cottage cheese
- ❏ 32 oz. container low-fat plain Greek yogurt
- ❏ 1 small bag low-fat shredded cheddar cheese
- ❏ 1 small package provolone or cheddar
- ❏ 1 package crumbled feta cheese

## FROZEN

- ❏ 1 cup frozen strawberries

## MISCELLANEOUS

- ❏ Paprika
- ❏ Cumin
- ❏ Jar minced garlic
- ❏ Ginger powder
- ❏ Fresh cilantro
- ❏ Onion powder
- ❏ Paprika
- ❏ Salt
- ❏ Pepper
- ❏ Italian seasoning
- ❏ Dijon mustard
- ❏ 10 wooden skewer sticks
- ❏ Dried oregano
- ❏ Red pepper flakes
- ❏ Chili powder
- ❏ Low-sodium taco seasoning
- ❏ Sugar
- ❏ Sriracha

# RESOURCES

## Chapter One

"Heart Disease and Stroke Statistics—2019 Update: A Report from the American Heart Association." 2020. *Circulation* 141 (2). https://doi.org/10.1161/cir.0000000000000746.

Gao, Yumin, Nino Isakadze, Eamon Duffy, Qicong Sheng, Jie Ding, Zane T. MacFarlane, Yingying Sang, et al. 2022. "Secular Trends in Risk Profiles among Adults with Cardiovascular Disease in the United States." *Journal of the American College of Cardiology* 80 (2): 126–37. https://doi.org/10.1016/j.jacc.2022.04.047.

Gulati, Rajiv, Atta Behfar, Jagat Narula, Ardaas Kanwar, Amir Lerman, Leslie Cooper, and Mandeep Singh. 2020. "Acute Myocardial Infarction in Young Individuals." *Mayo Clinic Proceedings* 95 (1): 136–56. https://doi.org/10.1016/j.mayocp.2019.05.001.

Hayashi, Meiso, Wataru Shimizu, and Christine M. Albert. 2015. "The Spectrum of Epidemiology Underlying Sudden Cardiac Death." *Circulation Research* 116 (12): 1887–1906. https://doi.org/10.1161/circresaha.116.304521.

Mahmood, Syed S, Daniel Levy, Ramachandran S Vasan, and Thomas J Wang. 2014. "The Framingham Heart Study and the Epidemiology of Cardiovascular Disease: A Historical Perspective." *The Lancet* 383 (9921): 999–1008. https://doi.org/10.1016/s0140-6736(13)61752-3.

Westerman, Stacy, and Nanette K. Wenger. 2016. "Women and Heart Disease, the Underrecognized Burden: Sex Differences, Biases, and Unmet Clinical and Research Challenges." *Clinical Science* 130 (8): 551–63. https://doi.org/10.1042/cs20150586.

## Chapter Two

Deckers, Kay, Syenna H. J. Schievink, Maria M. F. Rodriquez, Robert J. van Oostenbrugge, Martin P. J. van Boxtel, Frans R. J. Verhey, and Sebastian Köhler. 2017. "Coronary Heart Disease and Risk for Cognitive Impairment or Dementia: Systematic Review and Meta-Analysis." Edited by Stephen D Ginsberg. *PLOS ONE* 12 (9): e0184244. https://doi.org/10.1371/journal.pone.0184244.

Doege, Corinna, Mark Luedde, and Karel Kostev. 2021. "Epilepsy Is Associated with an Increased Incidence of Heart Failure Diagnoses." *Epilepsy & Behavior* 125 (December): 108393. https://doi.org/10.1016/j.yebeh.2021.108393.

El Khoudary, Samar R. 2020. "Age at Menopause Onset and Risk of Cardiovascular Disease around the World." *Maturitas* 141 (November): 33–38. https://doi.org/10.1016/j.maturitas.2020.06.007.

Frøjd LA, Munkhaugen J, Moum T, Sverre E, Nordhus IH, Papageorgiou C, Dammen T. 2021. "Insomnia in patients with coronary heart disease: prevalence and correlates." *Journal of Clinical Sleep Medicine* 17 (5): 931–938. https://doi.org/10.5664/jcsm.9082.

Houri Levi, Esther, Abdulla Watad, Aaron Whitby, Shmuel Tiosano, Doron Comaneshter, Arnon D. Cohen, and Howard Amital. 2016. "Coexistence of Ischemic Heart Disease and Rheumatoid Arthritis Patients—a Case Control Study." *Autoimmunity Reviews* 15 (4): 393–96. https://doi.org/10.1016/j.autrev.2016.01.006.

Ingebrigtsen, Truls Sylvan, Jacob Louis Marott, Jørgen Vestbo, Børge Grønne Nordestgaard, and Peter Lange. 2020. "Coronary Heart Disease and Heart Failure in Asthma, COPD and Asthma-COPD Overlap." *BMJ Open Respiratory Research* 7 (1): e000470. https://doi.org/10.1136/bmjresp-2019-000470.

Javaheri, Sogol, and Susan Redline. 2017. "Insomnia and Risk of Cardiovascular Disease." *Chest* 152 (2): 435–44. https://doi.org/10.1016/j.chest.2017.01.026.

John, Holly, Tracey E Toms, and George D Kitas. 2011. "Rheumatoid Arthritis: Is It a Coronary Heart Disease Equivalent?" *Current Opinion in Cardiology* 26 (4): 327–33. https://doi.org/10.1097/hco.0b013e32834703b5.

Kaiafa, Georgia, Ilias Kanellos, Christos Savopoulos, Nikolaos Kakaletsis, George Giannakoulas, and Apostolos I. Hatzitolios. 2015. "Is Anemia a

New Cardiovascular Risk Factor?" *International Journal of Cardiology* 186 (May): 117–24. https://doi.org/10.1016/j.ijcard.2015.03.159.

Kurth, Tobias. 2007. "Associations between migraine and cardiovascular disease," *Expert Review of Neurotherapeutics.* 7 (9): 1097–1104. https://doi .org/10.1586/14737175.7.9.1097.

Loncar, G., Obradovic, D., Thiele, H., von Haehling, S., and Lainscak, M. 2021. "Iron deficiency in heart failure." *ESC Heart Failure* 8: 2368–2379. https://doi.org/10.1002/ehf2.13265.

Newson, Louise. 2018. "Menopause and Cardiovascular Disease." *Post Reproductive Health* 24 (1): 44–49. https://doi.org/10.1177/2053369 117749675.

Pérez-Rubio, Alberto, J. Alberto San Román, and José María Eiros Bouza. 2021. "Impacto de La Vacunación Antigripal Sobre La Enfermedad Cardiovascular." *Medicina Clínica* 157 (1): 22–32. https://doi.org/10.1016/j.medcli.2021.01.017.

Rosamond, W. 2004. "Are Migraine and Coronary Heart Disease Associated? An Epidemiologic Review." *Headache: The Journal of Head and Face Pain* 44: S5-S12. https://doi.org/10.1111/j.1526-4610.2004.04103.x.

Tajbakhsh, Amir, Seyed Mohammad Gheibi Hayat, Hajar Taghizadeh, Ali Akbari, Masoumeh inabadi, Amir Savardashtaki, Thomas P. Johnston, and Amirhossein Sahebkar. 2020. "COVID-19 and Cardiac Injury: Clinical Manifestations, Biomarkers, Mechanisms, Diagnosis, Treatment, and Follow Up." *Expert Review of Anti-Infective Therapy* 19 (3): 345–57. https://doi.org/10.1080/14787210.2020.1822737.

Valtorta, Nicole K, Mona Kanaan, Simon Gilbody, Sara Ronzi, and Barbara Hanratty. 2016. "Loneliness and Social Isolation as Risk Factors for Coronary Heart Disease and Stroke: Systematic Review and Meta-Analysis of Longitudinal Observational Studies." *Heart* 102 (13): 1009–16. https://doi.org/10.1136/heartjnl-2015-308790.

## Chapter Three

Anderson, Todd J, Jean Grégoire, Glen J Pearson, Arden R Barry, Patrick Couture, Martin Dawes, Gordon A Francis, et al. 2016. "2016 Canadian Cardiovascular Society Guidelines for the Management of Dyslipidemia for the Prevention of Cardiovascular Disease in the Adult." *The Canadian Journal of Cardiology* 32 (11): 1263–82. https://doi.org/10.1016/j.cjca.2016.07.510.

Eichstaedt, Johannes C., Hansen Andrew Schwartz, Margaret L. Kern, Gregory Park, Darwin R. Labarthe, Raina M. Merchant, Sneha Jha, et al. 2015. "Psychological Language on Twitter Predicts County-Level Heart Disease Mortality." *Psychological Science* 26 (2): 159–69. https://doi.org/10.1177/0956797614557867.

Gerstein, Hertzel C, Helen M Colhoun, Gilles R Dagenais, Rafael Diaz, Mark Lakshmanan, Prem Pais, Jeffrey Probstfield, et al. 2019. "Dulaglutide and Cardiovascular Outcomes in Type 2 Diabetes (REWIND): A Double-Blind, Randomised Placebo-Controlled Trial." *The Lancet* 394 (10193): 121–30. https://doi.org/10.1016/s0140 -6736(19)31149-3.

Golaszewski, Natalie M., Andrea Z. LaCroix, Job G. Godino, Matthew A. Allison, JoAnn E. Manson, Jennifer J. King, Julie C. Weitlauf, et al. 2022. "Evaluation of Social Isolation, Loneliness, and Cardiovascular Disease among Older Women in the US." *JAMA Network Open* 5 (2): e2146461–61. https://doi.org/10.1001/jamanetworkopen.2021.46461.

Humphrey, Linda L., Rongwei Fu, Kevin Rogers, Michele Freeman, and Mark Helfand. 2008. "Homocysteine Level and Coronary Heart Disease Incidence: A Systematic Review and Meta-Analysis." *Mayo Clinic Proceedings* 83 (11): 1203–12. https://doi.org/10.4065/83.11.1203.

Humphrey, Linda L., Rongwei Fu, David I. Buckley, Michele Freeman, and Mark Helfand. 2008. "Periodontal Disease and Coronary Heart Disease Incidence: A Systematic Review and Meta-Analysis." *Journal of General Internal Medicine* 23 (12): 2079–86. https://doi.org/10.1007 /s11606-008-0787-6.

Kolber, Michael R., and Cathy Scrimshaw. 2014. "Family History of Cardiovascular Disease." *Canadian Family Physician* 60 (11): 1016–16. https://www.cfp.ca/content/60/11/1016.long.

Hageman, Steven, Lisa Pennells, Francisco Ojeda, Stephen Kaptoge, Kari Kuulasmaa, Tamar de Vries, Zhe Xu, et al. 2021. "SCORE2 Risk Prediction Algorithms: New Models to Estimate 10-Year Risk of Cardiovascular Disease in Europe." *European Heart Journal* 42 (25): 2439–54. https://doi.org/10.1093/eurheartj/ehab309.

Paterson, D. Ian, Natasha Wiebe, Winson Y. Cheung, John R. Mackey, Edith Pituskin, Anthony Reiman, and Marcello Tonelli. 2022. "Incident Cardiovascular Disease among Adults with Cancer." *JACC: CardioOncology* 4 (1): 85–94. https://doi.org/10.1016/j.jaccao .2022.01.100.

Sniderman, Allan D., George Thanassoulis, Tamara Glavinovic, Ann Marie Navar, Michael Pencina, Alberico Catapano, and Brian A. Ference. 2019. "Apolipoprotein B Particles and Cardiovascular Disease." *JAMA Cardiology*, October. https://doi.org/10.1001/jamacardio .2019.3780.

Tamang, H. K., Timilsina, U. Singh ,K. P., Shrestha, S. Raman, R. K., Panta, P. Karna, P. Khadka, L. Dahal, C. 2014. "Apo B/Apo A-I Ratio is Statistically A Better Predictor of Cardiovascular Disease (CVD) than Conventional Lipid Profile: A Study from Kathmandu Valley, Nepal." *Journal of Clinical and Diagnostic Research* 8 (2): 34–36. https://doi.org / 10.7860/JCDR/2014/7588.4000.

Trinder, Mark, Kaavya Paruchuri, Sara Haidermota, Rachel Bernardo, Seyedeh Maryam Zekavat, Thomas Gilliland, James Januzzi, and Pradeep Natarajan. 2022. "Repeat Measures of Lipoprotein(A) Molar Concentration and Cardiovascular Risk." *Journal of the American College of Cardiology* 79 (7): 617–28. https://doi.org/10.1016/j.jacc.2021.11.055.

Valtorta, Nicole K, Mona Kanaan, Simon Gilbody, Sara Ronzi, and Barbara Hanratty. 2016. "Loneliness and Social Isolation as Risk Factors for Coronary Heart Disease and Stroke: Systematic Review and Meta-Analysis of Longitudinal Observational Studies." *Heart* 102 (13): 1009–16. https://doi.org/10.1136/heartjnl-2015-308790.

## Chapter Four

Bahorik, Amber L, Stacy A Sterling, Cynthia I Campbell, Constance Weisner, Danielle Ramo, and Derek D Satre. 2018. "Medical and Non-Medical Marijuana Use in Depression: Longitudinal Associations with Suicidal Ideation, Everyday Functioning, and Psychiatry Service Utilization." *Journal of Affective Disorders* 241: 8–14. https://doi.org /10.1016/j.jad.2018.05.065.

Behlke, Lauren M., Eric J. Lenze, and Robert M. Carney. 2020. "The Cardiovascular Effects of Newer Antidepressants in Older Adults and Those with or at High Risk for Cardiovascular Diseases." *CNS Drugs* 34 (11): 1133–47. https://doi.org/10.1007/s40263-020-00763-z.

Bridges, Ledetra, and Manoj Sharma. 2017. "The Efficacy of Yoga as a Form of Treatment for Depression." *Journal of Evidence-Based Complementary & Alternative Medicine* 22 (4): 1017–28. https://doi.org /10.1177/2156587217715927.

Carney, Robert M., James A. Blumenthal, Kenneth E. Freedland, Marston Youngblood, Richard C. Veith, Matthew M. Burg, Carol Cornell, et al. 2004. "Depression and Late Mortality after Myocardial Infarction in the Enhancing Recovery in Coronary Heart Disease (ENRICHD) Study." *Psychosomatic Medicine* 66 (4): 466–74. https://doi.org/10.1097/01.psy.0000133362.75075.a6.

Chen, Yu, Gloria Mark, and Sanna Ali. 2016. "Promoting Positive Affect through Smartphone Photography." *Psychology of Well-Being* 6 (1). https://doi.org/10.1186/s13612-016-0044-4.

Chi X, Bo A, Liu T, Zhang P and Chi I. 2018. "Effects of Mindfulness-Based Stress Reduction on Depression in Adolescents and Young Adults: A Systematic Review and Meta-Analysis." *Frontiers in Psychology* 21 (9):1034. https://doi.org/10.3389/fpsyg.2018.01034.

Clarke, Robert, Elsa Valdes-Marquez, Michael Hill, Joanne Gordon, Martin Farrall, Anders Hamsten, Hugh Watkins, and Jemma C Hopewell. 2018. "Plasma Cytokines and Risk of Coronary Heart Disease in the PROCARDIS Study." *Open Heart* 5 (1): e000807. https://doi.org/10.1136/openhrt-2018-000807.

Elovainio, Marko, Anna-Mari Aalto, Mika Kivimäki, Sami Pirkola, Jouko Sundvall, Jouko Lönnqvist, and Antti Reunanen. 2009. "Depression and C-Reactive Protein: Population-Based Health 2000 Study." *Psychosomatic Medicine* 71 (4): 423–30. https://doi.org/10.1097/psy.0b013e31819e333a.

Feingold, Daniel, and Aviv Weinstein. 2020. "Cannabis and Depression." *Cannabinoids and Neuropsychiatric Disorders*, December, 67–80. https://doi.org/10.1007/978-3-030-57369-0_5.

Firth, Joseph, Wolfgang Marx, Sarah Dash, Rebekah Carney, Scott B. Teasdale, Marco Solmi, Brendon Stubbs, et al. 2019. "The Effects of Dietary Improvement on Symptoms of Depression and Anxiety." *Psychosomatic Medicine* 81 (3): 265–80. https://doi.org/10.1097/psy.0000000000000673.

Frishman, William H, and Pam Grewall. 2000. "Serotonin and the Heart." *Annals of Medicine* 32 (3): 195–209. https://doi.org/10.3109/07853890008998827.

Garg PK, O'Neal WT, Diez-Roux AV, Alonso A, Soliman EZ, Heckbert S. 2019. "Negative Affect and Risk of Atrial Fibrillation: MESA." *Journal of the American Heart Association* 8 (1): e010603. https://doi.org/10.1161/JAHA.118.010603.

Ghiadoni, Lorenzo, Ann E. Donald, Mark Cropley, Michael J. Mullen, Gillian Oakley, Mia Taylor, Georgina O'Connor, et al. 2000. "Mental Stress Induces Transient Endothelial Dysfunction in Humans." *Circulation* 102 (20): 2473–78. https://doi.org/10.1161/01.cir.102.20.2473.

Glassman, Alexander H., and Shapiro, Peter A. 1998. "Depression and the Course of Coronary Artery Disease." *American Journal of Psychiatry*, January. 155 (1): 4–11. https://doi.org/10.1176/ajp.155.1.4.

Hare, D. L., S. R. Toukhsati, P. Johansson, and T. Jaarsma. 2013. "Depression and Cardiovascular Disease: A Clinical Review." *European Heart Journal* 35 (21): 1365–72. https://doi.org/10.1093/eurheartj/eht462.

Harshfield, Eric L., Lisa Pennells, Joseph E. Schwartz, Peter Willeit, Stephen Kaptoge, Steven Bell, Jonathan A. Shaffer, et al. 2020. "Association between Depressive Symptoms and Incident Cardiovascular Diseases." *JAMA* 324 (23): 2396–2405. https://doi.org/10.1001/jama.2020.23068.

Irwin, Michael R., Carmen Carrillo, Nina Sadeghi, Martin F. Bjurstrom, Elizabeth C. Breen, and Richard Olmstead. 2021. "Prevention of Incident and Recurrent Major Depression in Older Adults with Insomnia." *JAMA Psychiatry*, November. https://doi.org/10.1001/jamapsychiatry.2021.3422.

Jang HY, Kim JH, Song Y-K, Shin J-Y, Lee H-Y, Ahn YM, Oh JM and Kim I-W. 2020. "Antidepressant Use and the Risk of Major Adverse Cardiovascular Events in Patients Without Known Cardiovascular Disease: A Retrospective Cohort Study." *Frontiers in Pharmacology* 11:594474. https://doi.org/10.3389/fphar.2020.594474.

Kaptoge S, Di Angelantonio E, et al. 2010. "C-Reactive Protein Concentration and Risk of Coronary Heart Disease, Stroke, and Mortality: An Individual Participant Meta-Analysis." *The Lancet* 375 (9709): 132–40. https://doi.org/10.1016/s0140-6736(09)61717-7.

Katon, W.J., et al. 2004. "Cardiac risk factors in patients with diabetes mellitus and major depression." *Journal of General Internal Medicine* 19(12): 1192–1199. https://doi.org/10.1111/j.1525-1497.2004.30405.x.

Kim, Yun Gi, Kwang-No Lee, Kyung-Do Han, Kyu-Man Han, Kyongjin Min, Ha Young Choi, Yun Young Choi, Jaemin Shim, Jong-Il Choi, and Young-Hoon Kim. 2022. "Association of Depression with Atrial Fibrillation in South Korean Adults." *JAMA Network Open* 5 (1): e2141772–72. https://doi.org/10.1001/jamanetworkopen.2021.41772.

Kim, Jae Hyun, Yun-Kyoung Song, Ha Young Jang, Ju-Young Shin, Hae-Young Lee, Yong Min Ahn, Jung Mi Oh, and In-Wha Kim. 2020. "Major Adverse Cardiovascular Events in Antidepressant Users within Patients with Ischemic Heart Diseases: A Nationwide Cohort Study." *Journal of Clinical Psychopharmacology* 40 (5): 475–81. https://doi.org/10.1097/JCP.0000000000001252.

Kleiger, Robert E., J. Philip Miller, J. Thomas Bigger, and Arthur J. Moss. 1987. "Decreased Heart Rate Variability and Its Association with Increased Mortality after Acute Myocardial Infarction." *The American Journal of Cardiology* 59 (4): 256–62. https://doi.org/10.1016/0002-9149(87)90795-8.

Laghrissi-Thode, Fouzia, William R. Wagner, Bruce G. Pollock, Peter C. Johnson, and Mitchell S. Finkel. 1997. "Elevated Platelet Factor 4 and β-Thromboglobulin Plasma Levels in Depressed Patients with Ischemic Heart Disease." *Biological Psychiatry* 42 (4): 290–95. https://doi.org/10.1016/s0006-3223(96)00345-9.

Musselman, Dominique L., Dwight L. Evans, and Charles B. Nemeroff. 1998. "The Relationship of Depression to Cardiovascular Disease." *Archives of General Psychiatry* 55 (7): 580. https://doi.org/10.1001/archpsyc.55.7.580.

Musselman, Dominique L., Tomer A., Manatunga AK, et al. "Exaggerated Platelet Reactivity in Major Depression." 1996. *American Journal of Psychiatry* 153 (10): 1313–17. https://doi.org/10.1176/ajp.153.10.1313.

Nicholson, A., H. Kuper, and H. Hemingway. 2006. "Depression as an Aetiologic and Prognostic Factor in Coronary Heart Disease: A Meta-Analysis of 6362 Events among 146 538 Participants in 54 Observational Studies." *European Heart Journal* 27 (23): 2763–74. https://doi.org/10.1093/eurheartj/ehl338.

O'Donnell MJ, Xavier D, Liu L, et al. 2010. "Risk factors for ischaemic and intracerebral haemorrhagic stroke in 22 countries (the INTERSTROKE study): a case-control study." *The Lancet*, July 10, 376 (9735): 112–23. https://doi.org/10.1016/S0140-6736(10)60834-3.

Osimo, Emanuele F., Toby Pillinger, Irene Mateos Rodriguez, Golam M. Khandaker, Carmine M. Pariante, and Oliver D. Howes. 2020. "Inflammatory Markers in Depression: A Meta-Analysis of Mean Differences and Variability in 5,166 Patients and 5,083 Controls." *Brain, Behavior, and Immunity*, February. https://doi.org/10.1016/j.bbi.2020.02.010.

Pattisapu, Varun K., Hua Hao, Yunxian Liu, Trevor-Trung Nguyen, Amy Hoang, C. Noel Bairey Merz, and Susan Cheng. 2021. "Sex- and Age-Based Temporal Trends in Takotsubo Syndrome Incidence in the United States." *Journal of the American Heart Association* 10 (20). https://doi.org/10.1161/jaha.120.019583.

Rajan, Selina, Martin McKee, Sumathy Rangarajan, Shrikant Bangdiwala, Annika Rosengren, Rajeev Gupta, Vellappillil Raman Kutty, et al. 2020. "Association of Symptoms of Depression with Cardiovascular Disease and Mortality in Low-, Middle-, and High-Income Countries." *JAMA Psychiatry* 77 (10): 1052. https://doi.org/10.1001/jamapsychiatry.2020.1351.

Reangsing, Chuntana, Tanapa Rittiwong, and Joanne Kraenzle Schneider. 2020. "Effects of Mindfulness Meditation Interventions on Depression in Older Adults: A Meta-Analysis." *Aging & Mental Health* 25 (7): 1–10. https://doi.org/10.1080/13607863.2020.1793901.

Ridker, Paul M., Nader Rifai, Marc Pfeffer, Frank Sacks, Serge Lepage, and Eugene Braunwald. 2000. "Elevation of Tumor Necrosis Factor-α and Increased Risk of Recurrent Coronary Events after Myocardial Infarction." *Circulation* 101 (18): 2149–53. https://doi.org/10.1161/01.cir.101.18.2149.

Sapolsky, R. M. 2001. "Depression, Antidepressants, and the Shrinking Hippocampus." *Proceedings of the National Academy of Sciences* 98 (22): 12320–22. https://doi.org/10.1073/pnas.231475998.

Spieker LE, Hürlimann D, Ruschitzka F, et al. 2002. "Mental stress induces prolonged endothelial dysfunction via endothelin-A receptors." *Circulation*, June 18; 105 (24): 2817–20. https://doi.org/10.1161/01.CIR.0000021598.15895.34.

Van der Kooy K, van Hout H, Marwijk H, Marten H, Stehouwer C, Beekman A. 2007. "Depression and the risk for cardiovascular diseases: systematic review and meta analysis." *International Journal of Geriatric Psychiatry*, July 22 (7): 613–26. https://doi.org/10.1002/gps.1723.

Vikenes, K., Farstad, M. and Nordrehaug, J., 1999. "Serotonin Is Associated with Coronary Artery Disease and Cardiac Events." *Circulation*, August 3. 100 (5): 483–9. https://doi.org/10.1161/01.CIR.100.5.483.

Wei D, Janszky I, Fang F, Chen H, Ljung R, Sun J, et al. 2021. "Death of an offspring and parental risk of ischemic heart diseases: A population-based cohort study." *PLOS Medicine* 18 (9): e1003790. https://doi.org/10.1371/journal.pmed.1003790.

Williams, Redford B., Douglas A. Marchuk, Kishore M. Gadde, John C. Barefoot, Katherine Grichnik, Michael J. Helms, Cynthia M. Kuhn, et al. 2001. "Central Nervous System Serotonin Function and Cardiovascular Responses to Stress." *Psychosomatic Medicine* 63 (2): 300–305. https://doi.org/10.1097/00006842-200103000-00016.

Y-Hassan, S., Tornvall, P. 2018. "Epidemiology, pathogenesis, and management of takotsubo syndrome." *Clinical Autonomic Research* 28: 53–65. https://doi.org/10.1007/s10286-017-0465-z.

## Chapter Five

American Psychological Association. 2020. "Stress in America 2020." Apa.org. American Psychological Association. October 2020. https://www.apa.org/news/press/releases/stress/2020/report-october.

Babaie, Javad, Yousef Pashaei Asl, Bahman Naghipour, and Gholamreza Faridaalaee. 2021. "Cardiovascular Diseases in Natural Disasters; a Systematic Review": Archives of Academic Emergency Medicine 9 (1): e36–36. https://doi.org/10.22037/aaem.v9i1.1208.

Baker, Brian, Miney Paquette, John P. Szalai, Helen Driver, Tamara Perger, Karin Helmers, Brian O'Kelly, and Sheldon Tobe. 2000. "The Influence of Marital Adjustment on 3-Year Left Ventricular Mass and Ambulatory Blood Pressure in Mild Hypertension." *Archives of Internal Medicine* 160 (22): 3453–58. https://doi.org/10.1001/archinte.160.22.3453.

Chiang, J. J., Park, H., Almeida, D. M., Bower, J. E., Cole, S. W., Irwin, M. R., McCreath, H., Seeman, T. E., & Fuligni, A. J. 2019. "Psychosocial stress and C-reactive protein from mid-adolescence to young adulthood." *Health Psychology* 38 (3); 259–267. https://doi.org/10.1037/hea0000701.

Cohen, S., D. Janicki-Deverts, W. J. Doyle, G. E. Miller, E. Frank, B. S. Rabin, and R. B. Turner. 2012. "Chronic Stress, Glucocorticoid Receptor Resistance, Inflammation, and Disease Risk." *Proceedings of the National Academy of Sciences* 109 (16): 5995–99. https://doi.org/10.1073/pnas.1118355109.

Dekker, M. J. H. J., J. W. Koper, M. O. van Aken, H. A. P. Pols, A. Hofman, F. H. de Jong, C. Kirschbaum, J. C. M. Witteman, S. W. J. Lamberts, and H. Tiemeier. 2008. "Salivary Cortisol Is Related to Atherosclerosis of Carotid Arteries." *The Journal of Clinical*

*Endocrinology & Metabolism* 93 (10): 3741–47. https://doi.org/10.1210
/jc.2008-0496.

Girod JP, Brotman DJ. 2004. "Does altered glucocorticoid homeostasis
increase cardiovascular risk?" *Cardiovascular Research* 64 (2): 217–26.
https://doi.org/10.1016/j.cardiores.2004.07.006.

Grewen, Karen M., Susan S. Girdler, and Kathleen C. Light. 2005.
"Relationship Quality: Effects on Ambulatory Blood Pressure and
Negative Affect in a Biracial Sample of Men and Women." *Blood
Pressure Monitoring* 10 (3): 117–24. https://doi.org/10.1097/00126097
-200506000-00002.

Guimont C, Brisson C, Dagenais GR, et al. 2006. "Effects of job
strain on blood pressure: a prospective study of male and female
white-collar workers." *American Journal of Public Health* 96: 1436–1439.
https://doi.org/10.2105/AJPH.2004.057679.

Hackett, Ruth A., Mika Kivimäki, Meena Kumari, and Andrew
Steptoe. 2016. "Diurnal Cortisol Patterns, Future Diabetes, and
Impaired Glucose Metabolism in the Whitehall II Cohort Study." *The
Journal of Clinical Endocrinology & Metabolism* 101 (2): 619–25.
https://doi.org/10.1210/jc.2015-2853.

Jiao, Zhen, Socrates V. Kakoulides, John Moscona, Jabar Whittier,
Sudesh Srivastav, Patrice Delafontaine, and Anand Irimpen. 2012.
"Effect of Hurricane Katrina on Incidence of Acute Myocardial
Infarction in New Orleans Three Years after the Storm." *The American
Journal of Cardiology* 109 (4): 502–5. https://doi.org/10.1016/j.amjcard
.2011.09.045.

Johansen C, Feychting M, Møller M, et al. 2002. "Risk of severe
cardiac arrhythmia in male utility workers: a nationwide Danish
cohort study." *American Journal of Epidemiology* 156 (9): 857–61.
https://doi.org/10.1093/aje/kwf137.

Kelly, Shona J., and Mubarak Ismail. 2015. "Stress and Type 2
Diabetes: A Review of How Stress Contributes to the Development
of Type 2 Diabetes." *Annual Review of Public Health* 36 (1): 441–62.
https://doi.org/10.1146/annurev-publhealth-031914-122921.

Kloner, Robert A, Jonathan Leor, W. Kenneth Poole, and Rebecca
Perritt. 1997. "Population-Based Analysis of the Effect of the
Northridge Earthquake on Cardiac Death in Los Angeles County,
California." *Journal of the American College of Cardiology* 30 (5): 1174–80.
https://doi.org/10.1016/S0735-1097(97)00281-7.

Kumari, Meena, Jenny Head, and Michael Marmot. 2004. "Prospective Study of Social and Other Risk Factors for Incidence of Type 2 Diabetes in the Whitehall II Study." *Archives of Internal Medicine* 164 (17): 1873. https://doi.org/10.1001/archinte.164.17.1873.

Lee, Sunmin, Graham A Colditz, Lisa F Berkman, and Ichiro Kawachi. 2003. "Caregiving and Risk of Coronary Heart Disease in U.S. Women." *American Journal of Preventive Medicine* 24 (2): 113–19. https://doi.org/10.1016/s0749-3797(02)00582-2.

Markovitz, Jerome H., Karen A. Matthews, Mary Whooley, Cora E. Lewis, and Kurt J. Greenlund. 2004. "Increases in Job Strain Are Associated with Incident Hypertension in the CARDIA Study." *Annals of Behavioral Medicine* 28 (1): 4–9. https://doi.org/10.1207/s15324796abm2801_2.

Matthews, Karen A., and Brooks B. Gump. 2002. "Chronic Work Stress and Marital Dissolution Increase Risk of Posttrial Mortality in Men from the Multiple Risk Factor Intervention Trial." *Archives of Internal Medicine* 162 (3): 309. https://doi.org/10.1001/archinte.162.3.309.

Mefford, Matthew, Murray Mittleman, Bonnie Li, Lei Qian, Kristi Reynolds, Hui Zhou, Teresa Harrison, et al. 2020. "Sociopolitical Stress and Acute Cardiovascular Disease Hospitalizations around the 2016 Presidential Election." *Proceedings of the National Academy of Sciences* 117 (43): 27054–27058. https://doi.org/10.1073/pnas.2012096117.

Mittleman, Murray A., and Elizabeth Mostofsky. 2011. "Physical, Psychological and Chemical Triggers of Acute Cardiovascular Events." *Circulation* 124 (3): 346–54. https://doi.org/10.1161/circulationaha.110.968776.

Nanayakkara, Natalie, Andrea J. Curtis, Stephane Heritier, Adelle M. Gadowski, Meda E. Pavkov, Timothy Kenealy, David R. Owens, et al. 2021. "Impact of Age at Type 2 Diabetes Mellitus Diagnosis on Mortality and Vascular Complications: Systematic Review and Meta-Analyses." *Diabetologia* 64 (2): 275–87. https://doi.org/10.1007/s00125-020-05319-w.

Raghavan, Sridharan, Jason L. Vassy, Yuk-Lam Ho, Rebecca J. Song, David R. Gagnon, Kelly Cho, Peter W. F. Wilson, and Lawrence S. Phillips. 2019. "Diabetes Mellitus–Related All-Cause and Cardiovascular Mortality in a National Cohort of Adults." *Journal of the American Heart Association* 8 (4). https://doi.org/10.1161/jaha.118.011295.

Rosengren, Annika, Steven Hawken, Stephanie Ôunpuu, Karen Sliwa, Mohammad Zubaid, Wael A Almahmeed, Kathleen Ngu Blackett, Chitr Sitthi-amorn, Hiroshi Sato, and Salim Yusuf. 2004. "Association of Psychosocial Risk Factors with Risk of Acute Myocardial Infarction in 11 119 Cases and 13 648 Controls from 52 Countries (the INTERHEART Study): Case-Control Study." *The Lancet* 364 (9438): 953–62. https://doi.org/10.1016/s0140-6736(04)17019-0.

Sharma, Ashish, Kameshwar Prasad, M.V. Padma, Manjari Tripathi, Rohit Bhatia, Mamta Bhusan Singh, and Anupriya Sharma. 2015. "Prevalence of Triggering Factors in Acute Stroke: Hospital-Based Observational Cross-Sectional Study." *Journal of Stroke and Cerebrovascular Diseases* 24 (2): 337–47. https://doi.org/10.1016/j.jstrokecerebrovasdis.2014.08.033.

Spruill, Tanya M. 2010. "Chronic Psychosocial Stress and Hypertension." *Current Hypertension Reports* 12 (1): 10–16. https://doi.org/10.1007/s11906 -009-0084-8.

Vaccarino, Viola, Zakaria Almuwaqqat, Jeong Hwan Kim, Muhammad Hammadah, Amit J. Shah, Yi-An Ko, Lisa Elon, et al. 2021. "Association of Mental Stress–Induced Myocardial Ischemia with Cardiovascular Events in Patients with Coronary Heart Disease." *JAMA* 326 (18): 1818–28. https://doi.org/10.1001/jama.2021.17649.

## Chapter 6

Alexander, Dominik D., Paula E. Miller, Ashley J. Vargas, Douglas L. Weed, and Sarah S. Cohen. 2016. "Meta-Analysis of Egg Consumption and Risk of Coronary Heart Disease and Stroke." *Journal of the American College of Nutrition* 35 (8): 704–16. https://doi.org/10.1080 /07315724.2016.1152928.

Appel, Lawrence J., Thomas J. Moore, Eva Obarzanek, William M. Vollmer, Laura P. Svetkey, Frank M. Sacks, George A. Bray, et al. 1997. "A Clinical Trial of the Effects of Dietary Patterns on Blood Pressure." *New England Journal of Medicine* 336 (16): 1117–24. https://doi.org/10 .1056/nejm199704173361601.

Aune, Dagfinn, NaNa Keum, Edward Giovannucci, Lars T Fadnes, Paolo Boffetta, Darren C Greenwood, Serena Tonstad, Lars J Vatten, Elio Riboli, and Teresa Norat. 2016. "Whole Grain Consumption and Risk of Cardiovascular Disease, Cancer, and All Cause and Cause Specific Mortality: Systematic Review and Dose-Response Meta-

Analysis of Prospective Studies." *BMJ*, June, i2716. https://doi.org /10.1136/bmj.i2716.

Becerra-Tomás, Nerea, Indira Paz-Graniel, Cyril W.C. Kendall, Hana Kahleova, Dario Rahelić, John L Sievenpiper, and Jordi Salas-Salvadó. 2019. "Nut Consumption and Incidence of Cardiovascular Diseases and Cardiovascular Disease Mortality: A Meta-Analysis of Prospective Cohort Studies." *Nutrition Reviews* 77 (10): 691–709. https://doi.org /10.1093/nutrit/nuz042.

Bibbins-Domingo, Kirsten, Glenn M. Chertow, Pamela G. Coxson, Andrew Moran, James M. Lightwood, Mark J. Pletcher, and Lee Goldman. 2010. "Projected Effect of Dietary Salt Reductions on Future Cardiovascular Disease." *New England Journal of Medicine* 362 (7): 590–99. https://doi.org/10.1056/nejmoa0907355.

Bonaccio M, Di Castelnuovo A, Costanzo S, et al. 2021. "Ultra-processed food consumption is associated with increased risk of all-cause and cardiovascular mortality in the Moli-sani Study." *The American Journal of Clinical Nutrition* 113 (2): 446–455. https://doi.org /10.1093/ajcn/nqaa299.

Estruch, Ramón, Emilio Ros, Jordi Salas-Salvadó, Maria-Isabel Covas, Dolores Corella, Fernando Arós, Enrique Gómez-Gracia, et al. 2013. "Primary Prevention of Cardiovascular Disease with a Mediterranean Diet." *New England Journal of Medicine* 368 (14): 1279–90. https://doi.org /10.1056/nejmoa1200303.

Guasch-Ferré, Marta, Yanping Li, Walter C. Willett, Qi Sun, Laura Sampson, Jordi Salas-Salvadó, Miguel A. Martínez-González, Meir J. Stampfer, and Frank B. Hu. 2022. "Consumption of Olive Oil and Risk of Total and Cause-Specific Mortality among U.S. Adults." *Journal of the American College of Cardiology* 79 (2): 101–12. https://doi.org/10.1016 /j.jacc.2021.10.041.

Hall, Kevin D., Alexis Ayuketah, Robert Brychta, Hongyi Cai, Thomas Cassimatis, Kong Y. Chen, Stephanie T. Chung, et al. 2019. "Ultra-Processed Diets Cause Excess Calorie Intake and Weight Gain: An Inpatient Randomized Controlled Trial of Ad Libitum Food Intake." *Cell Metabolism* 30 (1): 226. https://doi.org/10.1016/j.cmet.2019.05.020.

He, Jiang. 1999. "Dietary Sodium Intake and Subsequent Risk of Cardiovascular Disease in Overweight Adults." *JAMA* 282 (21): 2027. https://doi.org/10.1001/jama.282.21.2027.

Hu, Frank B. 1999. "A Prospective Study of Egg Consumption and Risk of Cardiovascular Disease in Men and Women." *JAMA* 281 (15): 1387. https://doi.org/10.1001/jama.281.15.1387.

Juul, Filippa, Niyati Parekh, Euridice Martinez-Steele, Carlos Augusto Monteiro, and Virginia W Chang. 2021. "Ultra-Processed Food Consumption among US Adults from 2001 to 2018." *The American Journal of Clinical Nutrition*, October. https://doi.org/10.1093/ajcn/nqab305.

Kraus, William E, Manjushri Bhapkar, Kim M Huffman, Carl F Pieper, Sai Krupa Das, Leanne M Redman, Dennis T Villareal, et al. 2019. "2 Years of Calorie Restriction and Cardiometabolic Risk (CALERIE): Exploratory Outcomes of a Multicentre, Phase 2, Randomised Controlled Trial." *The Lancet Diabetes & Endocrinology* 7 (9): 673–83. https://doi.org/10.1016/s2213-8587(19)30151-2.

Lichtenstein, Alice H., Lawrence J. Appel, Maya Vadiveloo, Frank B. Hu, Penny M. Kris-Etherton, Casey M. Rebholz, Frank M. Sacks, Anne N. Thorndike, Linda Van Horn, and Judith Wylie-Rosett. 2021. "2021 Dietary Guidance to Improve Cardiovascular Health: A Scientific Statement from the American Heart Association." *Circulation* 144 (23). https://doi.org/10.1161/cir.0000000000001031.

Ma, Yuan, Feng J. He, Qi Sun, Changzheng Yuan, Lyanne M. Kieneker, Gary C. Curhan, Graham A. MacGregor, et al. 2022. "24-Hour Urinary Sodium and Potassium Excretion and Cardiovascular Risk." *New England Journal of Medicine* 386 (3): 252–63. https://doi.org/10.1056/nejmoa2109794.

Mukamal, Kenneth J., Chiung M. Chen, Sowmya R. Rao, and Rosalind A. Breslow. 2010. "Alcohol Consumption and Cardiovascular Mortality among U.S. Adults, 1987 to 2002." *Journal of the American College of Cardiology* 55 (13): 1328–35. https://doi.org/10.1016/j.jacc.2009.10.056.

Narain, A., C. S. Kwok, and M. A. Mamas. 2016. "Soft Drinks and Sweetened Beverages and the Risk of Cardiovascular Disease and Mortality: A Systematic Review and Meta-Analysis." *International Journal of Clinical Practice* 70 (10): 791–805. https://doi.org/10.1111/ijcp.12841.

Pietinen, Pirjo, Erkki Vartiainen, Ritva Seppänen, Antti Aro, and Pekka Puska. 1996. "Changes in Diet in Finland from 1972 to 1992: Impact on Coronary Heart Disease Risk." *Preventive Medicine* 25 (3): 243–50. https://doi.org/10.1006/pmed.1996.0053.

Popkin, Barry M, and Corinna Hawkes. 2016. "Sweetening of the Global Diet, Particularly Beverages: Patterns, Trends, and Policy

Responses." *The Lancet Diabetes & Endocrinology* 4 (2): 174–86. https://doi.org/10.1016/s2213-8587(15)00419-2.

Sawicki, Caleigh M, Paul F Jacques, Alice H Lichtenstein, Gail T Rogers, Jiantao Ma, Edward Saltzman, and Nicola M McKeown. 2021. "Whole- and Refined-Grain Consumption and Longitudinal Changes in Cardiometabolic Risk Factors in the Framingham Offspring Cohort." *The Journal of Nutrition* 151 (9): 2790–99. https://doi.org/10.1093/jn/nxab177.

Srour, Bernard, Léopold K Fezeu, Emmanuelle Kesse-Guyot, Benjamin Allès, Caroline Méjean, Roland M Andrianasolo, Eloi Chazelas, et al. 2019. "Ultra-Processed Food Intake and Risk of Cardiovascular Disease: Prospective Cohort Study (NutriNet-Santé)." *BMJ* 365 (May): l1451. https://doi.org/10.1136/bmj.l1451.

Varady, Krista A., Sofia Cienfuegos, Mark Ezpeleta, and Kelsey Gabel. 2022. "Clinical Application of Intermittent Fasting for Weight Loss: Progress and Future Directions." *Nature Reviews Endocrinology*, February. https://doi.org/10.1038/s41574-022-00638-x.

Viguiliouk, Effie, Andrea J Glenn, Stephanie K Nishi, Laura Chiavaroli, Maxine Seider, Tauseef Khan, Marialaura Bonaccio, et al. 2019. "Associations between Dietary Pulses Alone or with Other Legumes and Cardiometabolic Disease Outcomes: An Umbrella Review and Updated Systematic Review and Meta-Analysis of Prospective Cohort Studies." *Advances in Nutrition* 10 (Supplement_4): S308–19. https://doi.org/10.1093/advances/nmz113.

Wang, Dong D., Yanping Li, Shilpa N. Bhupathiraju, Bernard A. Rosner, Qi Sun, Edward L. Giovannucci, Eric B. Rimm, et al. 2021. "Fruit and Vegetable Intake and Mortality: Results from 2 Prospective Cohort Studies of US Men and Women and a Meta-Analysis of 26 Cohort Studies." *Circulation* 143 (17). https://doi.org/10.1161/circulationaha.120.048996.

Wang, Xia, Xinying Lin, Ying Y Ouyang, Jun Liu, Gang Zhao, An Pan, and Frank B Hu. 2015. "Red and Processed Meat Consumption and Mortality: Dose–Response Meta-Analysis of Prospective Cohort Studies." *Public Health Nutrition* 19 (05): 893–905. https://doi.org/10.1017/s1368980015002062.

Whelton, Paul K. 1992. "The Effects of Nonpharmacologic Interventions on Blood Pressure of Persons with High Normal Levels." *JAMA* 267 (9): 1213. https://doi.org/10.1001/jama.1992.03480090061028.

Yang, Quanhe, Zefeng Zhang, Edward W Gregg, W Dana Flanders, Robert Merritt, and Frank B Hu. 2014. "Added Sugar Intake and Cardiovascular Diseases Mortality among US Adults." *JAMA Internal Medicine* 174 (4): 516–24. https://doi.org/10.1001/jamainternmed.2013.13563.

Zhang, Bo, Ke Xiong, Jing Cai, and Aiguo Ma. 2020. "Fish Consumption and Coronary Heart Disease: A Meta-Analysis." *Nutrients* 12 (8): 2278. https://doi.org/10.3390/nu12082278.

## Chapter Seven

Carpio-Rivera, Elizabeth, José Moncada-Jiménez, Walter Salazar-Rojas, and Andrea Solera-Herrera. 2016. "Acute Effects of Exercise on Blood Pressure: A Meta-Analytic Investigation." *Arquivos Brasileiros de Cardiologia* 106 (5). https://doi.org/10.5935/abc.20160064.

Centers for Disease Control and Prevention. National Diabetes Statistics Report, 2020. Atlanta, GA: Centers for Disease Control and Prevention, U.S. Dept of Health and Human Services; 2020.

Colberg, Sheri R., Ronald J. Sigal, Jane E. Yardley, Michael C. Riddell, David W. Dunstan, Paddy C. Dempsey, Edward S. Horton, Kristin Castorino, and Deborah F. Tate. 2016. "Physical Activity/Exercise and Diabetes: A Position Statement of the American Diabetes Association." *Diabetes Care* 39 (11): 2065–79. https://doi.org/10.2337/dc16-1728.

Einarson, Thomas R., Annabel Acs, Craig Ludwig, and Ulrik H. Panton. 2018. "Prevalence of Cardiovascular Disease in Type 2 Diabetes: A Systematic Literature Review of Scientific Evidence from across the World in 2007–2017." *Cardiovascular Diabetology* 17 (1). https://doi.org/10.1186/s12933-018-0728-6.

Howden, Erin J., Satyam Sarma, Justin S. Lawley, Mildred Opondo, William Cornwell, Douglas Stoller, Marcus A. Urey, Beverley Adams-Huet, and Benjamin D. Levine. 2018. "Reversing the Cardiac Effects of Sedentary Aging in Middle Age—a Randomized Controlled Trial." *Circulation* 137 (15): 1549–60. https://doi.org/10.1161/circulationaha.117.030617.

Islam, Mohammad R., Sophia Valaris, Michael F. Young, Erin B. Haley, Renhao Luo, Sabrina F. Bond, Sofia Mazuera, et al. 2021. "Exercise Hormone Irisin Is a Critical Regulator of Cognitive Function." *Nature Metabolism* 3 (8): 1058–70. https://doi.org/10.1038/s42255-021-00438-z.

Kamada, Masamitsu, Eric J. Shiroma, Julie E. Buring, Motohiko Miyachi, and I-Min Lee. 2017. "Strength Training and All-Cause, Cardiovascular Disease, and Cancer Mortality in Older Women: A Cohort Study." *Journal of the American Heart Association* 6 (11). https://doi.org/10.1161/jaha.117.007677.

Kraus, William E, Joseph A Houmard, Brian D Duscha, Kenneth J Knetzger, Michelle B Wharton, Jennifer S McCartney, Connie W Bales, et al. 2002. "Effects of the Amount and Intensity of Exercise on Plasma Lipoproteins." *The New England Journal of Medicine* 347 (19): 1483–92. https://doi.org/10.1056/NEJMoa020194.

Magkos, Faidon, Yannis Tsekouras, Stavros A. Kavouras, Bettina Mittendorfer, and Labros S. Sidossis. 2007. "Improved Insulin Sensitivity after a Single Bout of Exercise Is Curvilinearly Related to Exercise Energy Expenditure." *Clinical Science* 114 (1): 59–64. https://doi.org/10.1042/cs20070134.

Nanayakkara, Natalie, Andrea J. Curtis, Stephane Heritier, Adelle M. Gadowski, Meda E. Pavkov, Timothy Kenealy, David R. Owens, et al. 2021. "Impact of Age at Type 2 Diabetes Mellitus Diagnosis on Mortality and Vascular Complications: Systematic Review and Meta-Analyses." *Diabetologia* 64 (2): 275–87. https://doi.org/10.1007/s00125-020-05319-w.

Paoli, Antonio, Quirico F Pacelli, Tatiana Moro, Giuseppe Marcolin, Marco Neri, Giuseppe Battaglia, Giuseppe Sergi, Francesco Bolzetta, and Antonino Bianco. 2013. "Effects of High-Intensity Circuit Training, Low-Intensity Circuit Training and Endurance Training on Blood Pressure and Lipoproteins in Middle-Aged Overweight Men." *Lipids in Health and Disease* 12 (1). https://doi.org/10.1186/1476-511x-12-131.

Piercy, Katrina L., Richard P. Troiano, Rachel M. Ballard, Susan A. Carlson, Janet E. Fulton, Deborah A. Galuska, Stephanie M. George, and Richard D. Olson. 2018. "The Physical Activity Guidelines for Americans." *JAMA* 320 (19): 2020. https://doi.org/10.1001/jama.2018.14854.

Ramakrishnan, Rema, Aiden Doherty, Karl Smith-Byrne, Kazem Rahimi, Derrick Bennett, Mark Woodward, Rosemary Walmsley, and Terence Dwyer. 2021. "Accelerometer Measured Physical Activity and the Incidence of Cardiovascular Disease: Evidence from the UK Biobank Cohort Study." Edited by Amanda Paluch. *PLOS Medicine* 18 (1): e1003487. https://doi.org/10.1371/journal.pmed.1003487.

Reynolds, Andrew N., Jim I. Mann, Sheila Williams, and Bernard J. Venn. 2016. "Advice to Walk after Meals Is More Effective for Lowering Postprandial Glycaemia in Type 2 Diabetes Mellitus than Advice That Does Not Specify Timing: A Randomised Crossover Study." *Diabetologia* 59 (12): 2572–78. https://doi.org/10.1007/s00125-016-4085-2.

Tanasescu, Mihaela. 2002. "Exercise Type and Intensity in Relation to Coronary Heart Disease in Men." *JAMA* 288 (16): 1994. https://doi.org/10.1001/jama.288.16.1994.

Tian, Danyang, and Jinqi Meng. 2019. "Exercise for Prevention and Relief of Cardiovascular Disease: Prognoses, Mechanisms, and Approaches." *Oxidative Medicine and Cellular Longevity*. April 9, 2019. https://www.hindawi.com/journals/omcl/2019/3756750/.

Zhao, Min, Sreenivas P Veeranki, Costan G Magnussen, and Bo Xi. 2020. "Recommended Physical Activity and All Cause and Cause Specific Mortality in US Adults: Prospective Cohort Study." *BMJ*, July, m2031. https://doi.org/10.1136/bmj.m2031.

## Chapter Eight

Anderson, James W, Michael H Davidson, Lawrence Blonde, W Virgil Brown, W James Howard, Henry Ginsberg, Lisa D Allgood, and Kurt W Weingand. 2000. "Long-Term Cholesterol-Lowering Effects of Psyllium as an Adjunct to Diet Therapy in the Treatment of Hypercholesterolemia." *The American Journal of Clinical Nutrition* 71 (6): 1433–38. https://doi.org/10.1093/ajcn/71.6.1433.

Bernasconi, Aldo A., Michelle M. Wiest, Carl J. Lavie, Richard V. Milani, and Jari A. Laukkanen. 2020. "Effect of Omega-3 Dosage on Cardiovascular Outcomes." *Mayo Clinic Proceedings*, September. https://doi.org/10.1016/j.mayocp.2020.08.034.

Bjelakovic, Goran, Dimitrinka Nikolova, Lise Lotte Gluud, Rosa G Simonetti, and Christian Gluud. 2012. "Antioxidant Supplements for Prevention of Mortality in Healthy Participants and Patients with Various Diseases." *Cochrane Database of Systematic Reviews*, March. https://doi.org/10.1002/14651858.cd007176.pub2.

Burt, Lauren A., Emma O. Billington, Marianne S. Rose, Duncan A. Raymond, David A. Hanley, and Steven K. Boyd. 2019. "Effect of High-Dose Vitamin D Supplementation on Volumetric Bone Density and

Bone Strength." *JAMA* 322 (8): 736. https://doi.org/10.1001/jama
.2019.11889.

Danik, Jacqueline S., and JoAnn E. Manson. 2012. "Vitamin D and
Cardiovascular Disease." *Current Treatment Options in Cardiovascular
Medicine* 14 (4): 414–24. https://doi.org/10.1007/s11936-012-0183-8.

Mangione, Carol M., Michael J. Barry, Wanda K. Nicholson, Michael
Cabana, David Chelmow, Tumaini Rucker Coker, Esa M. Davis, et
al. 2022. "Vitamin, Mineral, and Multivitamin Supplementation to
Prevent Cardiovascular Disease and Cancer." *JAMA* 327 (23): 2326.
https://doi.org/10.1001/jama.2022.8970.

Rosique-Esteban, Nuria, Marta Guasch-Ferré, Pablo Hernández-
Alonso, and Jordi Salas-Salvadó. 2018. "Dietary Magnesium and
Cardiovascular Disease: A Review with Emphasis in Epidemiological
Studies." *Nutrients* 10 (2): 168. https://doi.org/10.3390/nu10020168.

Sunkara, Anusha, and Albert Raizner. 2019. "Supplemental Vitamins
and Minerals for Cardiovascular Disease Prevention and Treatment."
*Methodist DeBakey Cardiovascular Journal* 15 (3): 179–84. https://doi.org
/10.14797/mdcj-15-3-179.

Varshney, Ravi, and Matthew J Budoff. 2016. "Garlic and Heart
Disease." *The Journal of Nutrition* 146 (2): 416S421S. https://doi.org
/10.3945/jn.114.202333.

Zhang, Dongdong, Cheng Cheng, Yan Wang, Hualei Sun, Songcheng
Yu, Yuan Xue, Yiming Liu, Wenjie Li, and Xing Li. 2020. "Effect
of Vitamin D on Blood Pressure and Hypertension in the General
Population: An Update Meta-Analysis of Cohort Studies and
Randomized Controlled Trials." *Preventing Chronic Disease* 17 (January).
https://doi.org/10.5888/pcd17.190307.

Zhang, Xi, Yufeng Li, Liana C. Del Gobbo, Andrea Rosanoff, Jiawei
Wang, Wen Zhang, and Yiqing Song. 2016. "Effects of Magnesium
Supplementation on Blood Pressure." *Hypertension* 68 (2): 324–33.
https://doi.org/10.1161/hypertensionaha.116.07664.

Zozina, Vladlena I., Serghei Covantev, Olga A. Goroshko, Liudmila
M. Krasnykh, and Vladimir G. Kukes. n.d. "Coenzyme Q10 in
Cardiovascular and Metabolic Diseases: Current State of the Problem."
*Current Cardiology Reviews* 14 (3): 164–74. Accessed September 4, 2022.
http://doi.org/10.2174/1573403X14666180416115428

## Chapter Nine

Gerstein, Hertzel C., Naveed Sattar, Julio Rosenstock, Chinthanie Ramasundarahettige, Richard Pratley, Renato D. Lopes, Carolyn S.P. Lam, et al. 2021. "Cardiovascular and Renal Outcomes with Efpeglenatide in Type 2 Diabetes." *New England Journal of Medicine* 385 (10): 896–907. https://doi.org/10.1056/nejmoa2108269.

Hermida, Ramón C, Juan J Crespo, Manuel Domínguez-Sardiña, Alfonso Otero, Ana Moyá, María T Ríos, Elvira Sineiro, et al. 2019. "Bedtime Hypertension Treatment Improves Cardiovascular Risk Reduction: The Hygia Chronotherapy Trial." *European Heart Journal,* ehz754. https://doi.org/10.1093/eurheartj/ehz754.

Laffin, Luke J., and George L. Bakris. 2018. "Has the Sun Set on Nighttime Dosing in Uncomplicated Hypertension?" *Hypertension* 72 (4): 836–38. https://doi.org/10.1161/hypertensionaha.118.11207.

Mansi, Ishak A., Matthieu Chansard, Ildiko Lingvay, Song Zhang, Ethan A. Halm, and Carlos A. Alvarez. 2021. "Association of Statin Therapy Initiation with Diabetes Progression." *JAMA Internal Medicine* 181 (12): 1562. https://doi.org/10.1001/jamainternmed.2021.5714.

Slomski, Anita. 2021. "Statin Use Is Associated with Diabetes Progression." *JAMA* 326 (21): 2120. https://doi.org/10.1001/jama.2021.21431.

Thakker, Divyesh, Sunita Nair, Amit Pagada, Vinayak Jamdade, and Anuradha Malik. 2016. "Statin Use and the Risk of Developing Diabetes: A Network Meta-Analysis." *Pharmacoepidemiology and Drug Safety* 25 (10): 1131–49. https://doi.org/10.1002/pds.4020.

# INDEX

JOHN WHYTE, MD, MPH, is a popular physician and writer who has been communicating to the public about health issues for nearly two decades.

In his role as chief medical officer of WebMD, Dr. Whyte leads efforts to develop and expand strategic partnerships that create meaningful change around important and timely public health issues. Before joining WebMD, Whyte served as the director of professional affairs and stakeholder engagement at the Center for Drug Evaluation and Research at the US Food and Drug Administration. Dr. Whyte worked with health-care professionals, patients, and patient advocates, providing them with a focal point for advocacy, enhanced two-way communication, and collaboration; and assisting them in navigating the FDA on issues concerning drug development, review, and drug safety. He also developed numerous initiatives to address diversity in clinical trials.

Dr. Whyte worked for nearly a decade as the chief medical expert and vice president, health and medical education, at Discovery Channel, the leading nonfiction television network. In this role, he developed, designed, and delivered educational programming that appealed to medical and lay audiences. This included television shows and online content that won more than fifty awards, including numerous Tellys, CINE Golden Eagles, and Freddies.

Whyte is a board-certified internist. He completed an internal medicine residency at Duke University Medical Center and earned a master of public health in health policy and management at Harvard University School of Public Health. Before arriving in Washington, DC, he was a health services research fellow at Stanford and attending physician in the department of medicine.